# YOGA FOR BEGINNERS

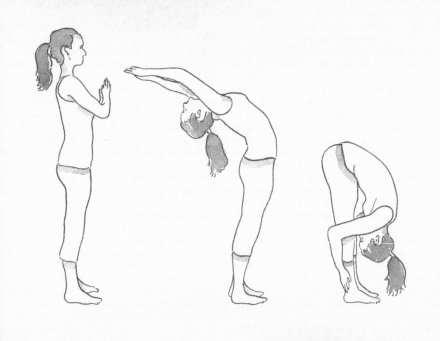

# YOGA
## FOR BEGINNERS

35 Simple Yoga Poses
to Calm Your Mind and
Strengthen Your Body

by CORY MARTIN

ROCKRIDGE
PRESS

# CONTENTS

# ACKNOWLEDGMENTS

A book is never written overnight or completed alone. I have been blessed with a team of teachers, editors, friends, and family who've made this all possible.

Thank you to Brian Hurley and the folks at Callisto Media for giving me the platform to combine my two biggest loves, writing and yoga. To all the others who contributed to this book, including Katy Brown and Tom Bingham, thank you for your hard work and dedication.

To the teachers who taught me how to be a yoga teacher: James Brown and Alexandria Crow, thank you for teaching me everything you know. I would not be qualified to write this book if it weren't for you. Nicole Sciacca, thank you for kicking my ass and being the first to say "you should become a teacher." Without your support I would still be the quiet girl in the back of the class.

To all the teachers who taught me how to put a sentence together: Mr. Boetel, Mr. Bird, Mrs. Watson, T.C. Boyle, and Aimee Bender, thank you for helping me to find my voice as a writer. To the teachers who taught me yoga when I was just a beginner: Meghan Kennedy Townsend, Elise Joan, David Romanelli, and Brock Cahill, thank you for your patience. Without your classes I never would have stuck with this practice.

To my Mom and Dad, thank you for always encouraging me to do the things I love, and supporting every crazy career idea I ever had. You taught me to follow my dreams and never give up. To my baby sister Cassie, thank you for willing to be my yoga guinea pig. Your constant feedback on my classes makes me a better teacher. To my Greg, thank you for reading early pieces of this book. Your unending support and love kept me typing away.

And finally, to all my students, thank you for trusting me to be your guide. Your smiling faces day in and day out are why I do what I do.

Namaste.

# PREFACE

I always thought of myself as a fairly athletic person. But my first yoga class? That was impossible. I struggled through every moment of it, dripped sweat all over my mat, and cursed inside my head, wondering how someone could become so attached to this stupid practice. It was physically demanding, and I was too worried about my quivering thighs and that acrobatic person on my left to feel any sense of calm.

But during the last five minutes of class, when I was lying on my back in the final resting pose, I finally understood the hype. Suddenly, my body relaxed. All the negative thoughts about yoga that were running through my head evaporated. Everything I had been fretting about disappeared. And I wondered: If I'm feeling this good after my very first try, what will happen if I keep coming back?

I went back to yoga the very next day, and for months after I continued to experiment with the practice. Over time that feeling I had at the end of my first class became more and more present in my daily life. And while that might sound all hippy-dippy, I promise you it's not. Yoga is about feeling good and making bright all the places in your life that seem dark. This is what yoga has provided to me over the years, and it's the reason I decided to become a yoga teacher.

I've been practicing yoga for over ten years, and I've taught in Los Angeles for nearly five. My students have met with me at small studios and exclusive gyms. I've instructed corporate clients on the beach and hundreds of others on the Santa Monica Pier. People of all shapes, sizes, and experience levels show up for my classes, and I lead them through a sequence of healthy, safe, mindful poses.

Some of my students show up to become enlightened, or at least less stressed. Others practice yoga to fit into their skinny jeans. Regardless of why someone practices yoga, I make it my mission to impart everything I know in a fun and approachable way. Sometimes we rock out to Led Zeppelin. Other times we practice yoga in complete silence.

Whether you want to learn the physical poses or you simply want to understand the philosophy behind the practice, you will find it all here. *Yoga for Beginners* is your guide, and I'm excited to be your teacher. As I say at the beginning of my classes, "This practice is all about you, so let's explore how yoga can fit into your life."

CHAPTER ONE

# BASICS

Now that you've met me, I think it's time to meet yoga. What is it? Where did it come from? What are its benefits? Is it a workout, or is it something else?

There are many aspects of yoga, and they might not all appeal to you. However, it helps to understand them in order to find the style of yoga that suits you best. For me, it started as a purely physical practice. Soon, it became a lifestyle. For you, it might be completely different. But that's the beauty of yoga: You decide how it should exist in your life. So let's get down to the basics.

# What Is Yoga?

Yoga is now. That's it. That's all there is to know. Good night and thank you.

Okay, it's far more than that. But that sentence, *Yoga is now*, is the whole thing boiled down to three words.

The problem is that "now" is a pretty hard concept to put into practice in our daily lives. Have you ever tried to live in the moment, right here, right now, with no distractions and no other thoughts in your head? It's difficult. That's why a man named Patanjali, who lived during the second century BC, wrote the *Yoga Sutras* as a guide to yoga. "Yoga is now" is the first of his 196 sutras. But it's only the beginning of his teachings.

Patanjali, who is considered to be the founder of the philosophy of yoga, defines yoga as the ability to cease identification with the movements of the mind—in other words, to "live in the now." The literal translation of *yoga* is "to yoke" or "union" or "to join." Modern yogis translate this as the union of the mind and the body. This is why when most of us think of yoga, we think of Down Dog or fancy balancing poses. Much of the work that we do in the physical practice of yoga is meant to carry over into our mental states.

For example, if we hold a pose and work through some discomfort in our thighs or our arms, then we learn to understand that when we are faced with the pain that comes from the difficult times in our lives, we have the strength to get through it. The physical helps the mental and vice versa; therefore, one cannot exist without the other, and that is why we have yoga—or the union of the two.

# The Eight Limbs of Yoga

Patanjali understood that there was more to yoga than just moving the body. Achieving the now is hard work. Using the lessons of his *Sutras,* he broke yoga down into the following eight areas or "limbs," known as *ashtanga*.

**YAMAS**

self-control

**NIYAMAS**

methods of discipline

**ASANAS**

physical postures

**PRANAYAMA**

breath work

**PRATYAHARA**

assistance with withdrawing from the senses

**DHARANA**

concentration

**DHYANA**

meditation

**SAMADHI**

absorption or liberation from the mind and the body

As you can see, yoga is more than just a kickass workout. *Asanas*—the physical postures—are just one part of the yoga practice. In order to comprehend yoga as a whole, we need to understand all eight of these principles.

I recognize that for now these Sanskrit terms probably mean nothing to you, and you might just want to move on to the poses. That's perfectly fine. However, if you begin to practice yoga in a yoga studio or start to follow videos online, it is inevitable that some of these Sanskrit words will come up in one or more of your classes. That is why I mention them here, so they will reveal themselves in ways that help you.

Besides asana, the most referenced of the branches of *ashtanga* are the first two principles: the *yamas* and *niyamas*. Patanjali breaks down each of these into five different areas, which are described below.

## Yamas

The *yamas* describe ways in which we can control our actions and our reactions. The five *yamas* are as follows:

1. *Ahimsa*

2. *Satya*

3. *Asteya*

4. *Brahmacharya*

5. *Aparigraha*

### AHIMSA

*Ahimsa* literally translates to "not injury." The easiest way to think about it is like the doctor's Hippocratic oath, which says, "First, do no harm." It is the guiding principle that physicians use in making any major medical decision. According to *ahimsa*, it should guide yoga practice as well.

This principle can be as simple as the lessons taught to kids, such as do not hit and do not fight, or it can get more complex in the form of exercising restraint. Examples of this are not talking ill of others or trying not to harbor hatred of those who have done wrong. But *ahimsa* doesn't solely apply to how to treat others. It applies to how you treat your own body as well. In a sense, it asks you to be your own doctor.

*Ahimsa* encourages you to consider the following issues:

✦ Preventing injury or sickness

✦ Learning to rest when you've overdone it

✦ Finding ways to cope with stress at work or home

Some yogis also translate *ahimsa* to being vegan and not harming animals. This works great for some, but not for all. Deciding what it means to do no harm to your body can be a personal matter.

## SATYA

*Satya* is the practice of honesty—not only with others but also with yourself. Being truthful is one of the biggest lessons that you can translate to the yoga mat. Once you start to learn the poses, how can you be honest with yourself? How can you listen to your body and understand when you've pushed it too far or not far enough? Practicing *satya* can help you feel better about yourself.

## ASTEYA

*Asteya* is the practice of not stealing. It can also mean not coveting the things that belong to others, whether they are material or intangible. It's the practice of letting go of jealous feelings and ceasing to compare yourself with others.

## BRAHMACHARYA

*Brahmacharya* is perhaps the most interesting *yama*. It has
been translated to mean abstinence, and Patanjali did believe
in celibacy. However, in today's modern world that might
not be possible, so we translate this one to mean "not spending your time on things that waste your energy." There are
plenty of examples of this. Perhaps you're always saying yes
to every invite you get and you're exhausted. Maybe you're
holding on to relationships that no longer serve you or the
other person. *Brahmacharya* urges you to rid your life of the
things that drain you.

## APARIGRAHA

*Aparigraha* means "nongreed." This *yama* encourages you
to stop living in excess. Have you ever had thoughts like,
"If I had more money, or a bigger house, or better clothes,
I would be happy"? *Aparigraha* encourages you to let go of
those thoughts and be content with what you do have. To
live by the principle of *Aparigraha*, do your best to derive
happiness from yourself and the love around you rather
than preferring things that you can buy or obtain.

## *Niyamas*

The *niyamas* consist of the following:

✦ *Saucha*

✦ *Santosha*

✦ *Tapas*

✦ *Svadhyaya*

✦ *Isvara Pranidhana*

These five concepts lay out ways to act in the world. They encourage you to contemplate how you act as an individual, consistently.

## SAUCHA
*Saucha* means "cleanliness." This can mean everything from keeping the house clean to eating pure and good foods to freeing your life of things that do not serve you. It's a simple concept and one that can relate to just about every aspect of your life.

## SANTOSHA
Translated as "contentment," *santosha* is all about being happy with where you are right now. It's still fine to have goals, but even as you strive for them, be content with what you have in the moment. Have aim and intention, but don't be fixated on the outcome.

## TAPAS
*Tapas* means "working through the difficult things in life in order to create change." Sometimes in class teachers will talk about building *tapas*, which can mean "heat." This heat is meant to create a literal change—perhaps by making you more flexible or stronger or leaner. In the general sense, however, it is about working through problems and find-ing solutions. You know that saying, "What doesn't kill you makes you stronger"? Well, whoever came up with it might have read a little bit about *tapas*.

## SVADHYAYA
*Svadhyaya* is the act of self-study. It asks you to become your own keeper. Through self-study you begin to learn which *tapas* are good for you, which pain is going to help you grow,

and which pain takes you away from the practice of *ahimsa* and causes harm. *Svadhyaya* concerns taking responsibility for your life and contemplating what you need to grow.

### ISVARA PRANIDHANA

*Isvara pranidhana* acknowledges that something "out there" is bigger than humanity as a whole. This principle emphasizes that individuals have no real control over anything, regardless of their belief systems.

## Asana

Asana is the physical practice of yoga. These are the poses, the Down Dogs and the Up Dogs, and all the stretching and balancing in between. Later, as you learn more about the physical practice, asana will help you grasp the other aspects of yoga.

## Pranayama

*Pranayama* is breath work. There are many types of yogic breathing out there, but one of the simplest is learning to breathe slowly and deeply. It is said that most people use only a small portion of their lungs' capacity to breathe. Making a conscious effort to fill your lungs with air can create a calming effect that relieves stress.

## Pratyahara

*Pratyahara* is the practice of withdrawing from the senses in order to focus in on your own thoughts, by being able to look inward. It's like sitting at your desk to work and turning off your phone and the Internet so that you don't get distracted.

## Dharana

*Dharana* is the ability to concentrate on one thing and let all else drift away. Think about a professional athlete, the golfer making that winning putt or the football player running that last touchdown. He or she is so focused on the task ahead that everything else disappears. This ability to concentrate intently leads to taking the next step—meditation.

## Dhyana

*Dhyana* is the practice of meditation. I have a teacher who describes meditation as being able to tune everything else out and focus on one thing. She prompts students to focus solely on their breath and when their minds start to wander to come back to the breath. This is the simplest way to meditate as discussed later in this book.

## Samadhi

*Samadhi* is the highest point of yoga. It's that perfect balance where the mind is calm and the body is in a state of internal stability. It is what all the other principles of yoga are designed to help us achieve. It is the ultimate "now."

# A Brief History of Yoga

We've touched on some of the history of yoga with Patanjali's sutras and the eight principles, but there is still so much to be known. How did this thing we call yoga come to be?

The history of yoga can be broken down into five periods:

1. Vedic

2. Pre-Classical

3. Classical

4. Post-Classical

5. Modern

## Vedic Yoga

The Vedic period of yoga spans the time of 500 to 1000 BC. It is during this period that the Rig Vedas were written. These books of hymns are the oldest known scriptures in existence, and they contain the early beginnings of yoga. Rather than emphasizing the postures, the Rig Vedas sought to join the material and spiritual worlds. Everything was based on the spiritual, and Vedic yogis were adept at focusing their minds for long periods of time. This focus produced visions that allowed the yogis to see the root of their very existence.

## Pre-Classical Yoga

The Pre-Classical period of yoga is marked by the publication of the *Upanishads*, which arrived somewhere between the fifth and seventeenth centuries BC. The *Upanishads* not only furthered the knowledge of the Rig Vedas, but also broke them down to explain the ultimate reality and the transcendental self. These became guides to explain how to apply the knowledge of the Rig Vedas to your daily life. Later during this period, the *Bhagavad Gita* was written. This text is the first book to be devoted entirely to yoga. It tells the story of the god Krishna and the solider Ardjuna. This parable introduces the idea of disassociating with the ego to avoid difficulties or pain. Today, many yogis reference this text to explain the letting go of the ego.

## Classical Yoga

This period centers around Patanjali's *Yoga Sutras* and the eight principles of yoga, which were discussed earlier in this chapter. This period produced the idea that the mind and body were separate and they must be worked on separately via meditation and asana.

## Post-Classical Yoga

During the Post-Classical period, yogi masters began to focus on the strengths and abilities of the body. They created a system of physical postures that would challenge the body and help prolong its life. This system of postures became Hatha yoga and is the beginning of the asana practice that we know today. It is here that yogis wrapped their minds around the concept of living in the moment. The purpose of the postures was to facilitate concentration and meditation to reach the state of *samadhi*, which is the highest mental state of yoga.

## Modern Yoga

In 1893, Swami Vivekananda came over from India to address the Parliament of Religions held in Chicago. It was there that yoga was first introduced to the American public and the Modern period of yoga began.

The Modern period emphasizes the asanas and efforts toward uniting the mind and the body. It draws from every previous period, focusing on works such as the *Bhagavad Gita* and Patanjali's *Yoga Sutras*. Today, teachers from all over the world work to spread the knowledge of yoga, and there are many different styles in existence.

# Styles of Yoga

While these styles of yoga all stem from the same historical roots, they are distinct in their focus and beliefs. Here are seven of the most popular styles:

- ✦ Ashtanga
- ✦ Kundalini
- ✦ Hatha
- ✦ Bikram
- ✦ Kriya
- ✦ Raja
- ✦ Iyengar

## Ashtanga Yoga

Not to be confused with Patanjali's eight-limbed path to yoga, Ashtanga Yoga is a system of yoga created by Sri K. Pattabhi Jois. It is known to be one of the most physically challenging versions of yoga. These series are to be practiced six days a week, except for moon days—days of the new and full moon—during which the practitioner will rest. The Ashtanga style is usually a self-practice. It is done under the Mysore style, which requires a teacher to assist the student into poses. Students discover when they are ready to move on to the next series, much like achieving different belts in karate. Ashtanga consists of six series, and very few people have made it to the final one.

## Kundalini Yoga

Kundalini was brought to the United States in 1968 by Yogi Bhajan. It's called the yoga of awareness and is considered the most spiritual practice that exists today. *Kundalini* refers to the energy that lies dormant at the base of the spine. Practicing meditation, breath work, mantra, dance, and asana raises this energy up the spine and out through the chakras. (A mantra is a chant that supports meditation. A chakra is a point of energy in the human body.) The goal of Kundalini is to create a sense of well-being and heightened awareness.

## Hatha Yoga

Hatha is the most widely practiced form of yoga, combining movement with conscious breathing. This system was developed by Yogi Swatmarama to develop strength and flexibility using a set of physical postures. These poses are meant to align the skin, muscles, and bones of the body.

## Bikram Yoga

Created by Bikram Choudhury, Bikram Yoga is a set
sequence of 26 postures and two breathing exercises. It
is meant to restore the body to its proper working order,
creating a sense of good health, proper weight, muscle tone,
and flexibility. Bikram Yoga is practiced under a strict set of
guidelines, which includes a room heated to 105 degrees
with 40 percent humidity. Only teachers who have trained
under Bikram can teach the Bikram method.

## Kriya Yoga

Kriya yoga is an ancient system brought to the West by
Paramahansa Yogananda. Kriya is a system of meditation
using breath, concentration, and a meditation technique
meant to accelerate one's spiritual growth. It focuses on
controlling the breath.

## Raja Yoga

Raja yoga is sometimes referred to as Royal yoga. It is known
as the yoga of the mind. The premise of the practice is this:
The mind controls the world. Controlling the mind makes it
possible to control the world around us. The biggest part of
the practice is meditation. Other techniques are included,
such as asana and breath work. These are meant to teach
practitioners to calm their minds and bring them to one
point of focus.

## Iyengar Yoga

Iyengar is based on the eight limbs of yoga described in
Patanjali's *Yoga Sutras*. Founded by BKS Iyengar in 1937,

Iyengar is a system of postures that focuses on alignment and breath control. It is a form of Hatha yoga that is characterized by its great attention to detail. Iyengar was one of the first teachers to use props in order to make yoga more accessible to everyone—beginners, advanced, seniors, those who are ill, and all others.

# What Yoga Can Bring to Your Life

According to the latest Yoga in America study conducted by Sports Marketing Surveys USA on behalf of *Yoga Journal* in 2012, there are 20.4 million Americans who practice yoga, and 44.8 percent of them consider themselves to be beginners. When asked in the survey why people are doing yoga, the top five reasons for starting were as follows:

1. Flexibility (78.3 percent)

2. General conditioning (62.2 percent)

3. Stress relief (59.6 percent)

4. To improve overall health (58.5 percent)

5. Physical fitness (55.1 percent)

I can tell you from my own experience that all five of these reasons are excellent and valid reasons to come to yoga. However, there is far more to be gained from yoga than strength, flexibility, good health, and less stress.

As one of the few forms of exercise that also focuses on the mental aspect of health, yoga's list of benefits is quite long. The following sections offer you a small sampling of what you can expect when you start to practice, but don't be surprised if you notice other changes happening as well.

## Increasing Your Sense of Space

Proprioception is the ability to understand how your body moves in space. It's me standing at the front of the room asking you to step your right foot forward and point your toes straight ahead. You do this without having to look down. By focusing on alignment in the poses, yogis' proprioception increases.

## Supporting Weight Loss

As a system of exercise that can increase your heart rate and build muscle, yoga inevitably makes weight loss possible. But one of the other benefits of yoga is that many people begin to eat more mindfully. Because they start to feel better overall, they start to make healthier choices for their bodies.

## Adding to Your Strength

The poses require you to hold your own body weight in a variety of ways. This stresses your muscles in a manner that encourages them to get stronger, much like lifting weights.

## Enhancing Flexibility

This is the obvious benefit that comes to mind when you think of yoga. Stick with the practice. You'll find that your joints become more mobile and you wake with less stiffness.

## Improving Balance

Many poses in the practice work on balance, but one of the major components of every pose is engaging the core muscles. Doing so teaches you to center your body and achieve physical balance with ease. This balance sometimes starts to transfer into our daily lives as well. So, you might also create a better work-life balance, too.

## Easing Stress

Yoga gives you the tools to relax, either through asana, breath work, or meditation. Breathing in a deep mindful manner calms the nervous system. The physical practice produces endorphins, and meditation brings clarity. (Endorphins are hormones that produce a feeling of well-being.)

## Perfecting Your Posture

Yoga strengthens the muscles of the core (generally, the abdomen and lower back), which causes your body to seek out a more proper upright position. It also keeps the spine supple and its surrounding muscles flexible.

## Improving Circulation

Yoga has many proven benefits for the heart, including lowering blood pressure and lowering heart rate. Also, the movement associated with yoga encourages the body's lymph fluid to drain more properly. Lymph contains the white blood cells in the human immune system.

## Enhancing Focus

One of the goals of yoga is to concentrate on the breath and the alignment of the postures. Doing so clears the mind of extraneous thoughts. By training the brain to focus like this on the mat, you are able to focus in your daily life.

## Assisting with Sleep

Clearly, you expend energy when you move your body and are therefore more tired at the end of the day. But because yoga also works on easing stress and creating focus, it becomes easier to slip off into slumber at night.

## Adding to Your Inner Strength

As your body gets stronger and more flexible, you tend to gain a confidence that you might not have had previously. Through *tapas* (the heat you create to initiate change), you might find that experiences in your life improve without you having made a conscious effort.

## Protecting Yourself from Injury

Because the asana practice of yoga focuses on strength and flexibility, many people will find that their bodies become stronger and more resistant to injury than they were prior to beginning yoga.

## Improving Athletic Performance

Yoga strengthens the body and makes athletes agile and strong. It also brings a new sense of clarity or focus to athletes that they can use to improve their performances. If you name a sport, I guarantee you can find someone who has created a system of yoga poses that will produce sport-specific results and prevent common injuries.

## Managing Chronic Conditions

Many different types of yoga have sprung up to help people deal with specific needs. There is pre- and post-natal yoga that helps expectant and new mothers adapt to the changes in their bodies. Yoga for the aging can help keep seniors active and free from injury. Yoga practice can also benefit those managing diseases such as diabetes or multiple sclerosis.

Regardless of your physical capabilities, if you have a desire to practice yoga, there is a way to do it. It's simply a matter of sorting through your options and finding a practice that works best for you to create the greatest array of benefits.

CHAPTER TWO

# PRACTICE

A saying has been popping up in the yoga world lately that sums it up perfectly: "practice, not perfection." In order to reap the benefits of practicing yoga, you have to put in the work, but your efforts don't have to be perfect. You simply need to commit to practicing yoga on a regular basis. But how do you *do* that? And what do you need? Here are some answers to these very good questions.

## Making a Commitment

The best way to practice yoga is regularly and often. However, this does not mean that you have to commit an hour and a half of your day to flowing through the poses. In fact if you have just one free minute a day, you can do yoga. Remember those eight principles of yoga?

1.  Self-control (*yamas*)

2.  Methods of discipline (*niyamas*)

3. Physical postures (asanas)

4. Breath work (*pranayama*)

5. Withdrawing from the senses (*pratyahara*)

6. Concentration (*dharana*)

7. Meditation (*dhyana*)

8. Meditative absorption or liberation from the mind and the body (*samadhi*)

This is where they come into play. Because yoga is more than a purely physical workout, you can find the time and space to practice some element of it every day. For example, do a simple breathing exercise where you spend a minute decompressing. Take five minutes to stretch out the tightness in your hips and shoulders from sitting at a desk all day. Practice an entire sequence that gets your heart pumping and your body moving. Maybe it's as easy as keeping your promise to practice one of the *yamas* like *santosha*, or contentment, for the day. No matter what form your commitment takes, the objective is to do yoga daily in order to maximize its benefits over time.

Here are a few simple ideas to help you commit to a regular practice:

SET ASIDE A SPECIFIC TIME EVERY DAY. Practice some form of yoga, whether it's meditating, breath work, a few poses, or a whole sequence of poses. Pick a time that you can commit to every day and stick to it. Set an alarm on your phone to remind you, put it in your calendar, leave a sticky note on your bathroom mirror. Do something to make the practice a part of your life.

**PUT YOUR MAT OUT AT NIGHT.** Seeing your mat in the morning can be a positive reinforcement. Set it next to your front door when you leave for work or go out for some other reason. That way, when you return home, your mat will be the first thing you see.

**REWARD YOURSELF FOR COMMITTING TO YOGA.** Perhaps you want a new mat or a new pair of yoga pants or you simply want a treat at your favorite restaurant. Set up a system that makes sense to you and reward yourself every week for committing to your practice.

**FIND A YOGA CHALLENGE ON SOCIAL MEDIA.** Look up the hashtags #yoga or #yogaeverydamnday to find teachers all over the world, then join a challenge that fits with your experience. These challenges will not only teach you new poses, but they also will hold you accountable for doing some form of yoga daily.

**SET AN INTENTION.** Ask yourself, "Why am I doing yoga?" Once you figure out the reason, remind yourself of it daily. Find something that inspires and encourages you to keep going. This can be a word, a quote, a mantra, or a goal. Find something positive that moves you and focus on it every time you come to the mat.

**FOCUS ON ONE OF THE *YAMAS* OR THE *NIYAMAS*.** Let it be your guide for the day or the week in all that you do. For example, if you pick *satya*, every time you make a decision to do something, wonder, *Am I being truthful? Am I being honest with myself and others?*

**LISTEN TO MUSIC.** There is something about good music that will get you up and moving. While this might not work if you intend to meditate, it will certainly get you off the couch and onto your mat if you're feeling lazy.

**GET A FRIEND TO JOIN YOU.** Maybe you can practice together every day. Perhaps you check in with each other to make sure you're keeping up with your practice. Whatever it is, find someone to keep you accountable.

**BE KIND TO YOURSELF.** Do not beat yourself up if you miss a day or you fail to meet one of your goals. Accept it for what it is and move on. Practice *ahimsa* (doing no harm) and remember "practice, not perfection."

Once you've committed to the practice, it is important to find a place where you feel comfortable doing yoga. Not everyone has empty rooms with nice bamboo floors like many yoga studios, so be ready to get creative with this.

# Clearing a Space

I live in Los Angeles, where rents are high and space is limited. Rentals seem to come with some form of an obligatory beige carpet. For the longest time I hated practicing at home because I never felt comfortable: The carpet was too squishy, I had to move my couch, and the lights in the living room were in my eyes. But then one day I got creative and decided to test out my galley kitchen. I laid out my mat on the linoleum floor and found that I could move with ease. Because some of the counters and cabinets stuck out at just the right heights, I was actually able to improve my practice by using these items as props. I share this story because I want you to know that no matter what your living situation is, I am certain that you can find a space that works for you.

Once you find this space, claim it as your yoga spot. Regardless of its dual purpose as a kitchen or your living room, take note that this is going to be your place of refuge. This is where you'll come to let go of your day, clear your mind, and move your body.

As you start to practice yoga, you begin to tune out the exterior world. Suddenly, the only things that matter are those that are on your mat. This is one of the benefits of the practice. If you can start to think of your yoga space as a special place, then when you step onto your mat, it will be that much easier to focus on what your body and mind are doing. It will be easier to let go of the things that do not serve you.

# Choosing Clothing

Now that you've got your yoga spot, what are you going to wear? Truthfully, if you're in the privacy of your own home and you want to wear your birthday suit, go for it. However, if you're looking for something a little more modest, certain fabrics and types of clothes are more suited to moving in and out of the poses than others. For example, big baggy T-shirts make yoga difficult. When you're in Down Dog and your head is toward the ground and your hips are lifted, guess where that shirt is going? Right over your face. Unless you're planning on doing yoga blindfolded, fitted tops are best because they allow you to move without distraction.

As for pants or shorts, there are plenty of options on the market. Because yoga has become such a big business, most brands and stores carry yoga clothes. When shopping, look for things that are comfortable. Then, try them on and move around. Here's a little test for pants. In the dressing room, bend at your hips and reach for your toes. If the pants stay up and they're not see-through, they'll work. If the waistband starts to creep toward your thighs and you can see your undergarments, look for a different pair. Men's pants tend to be a little looser and a little less transparent than women's. Again, try them on. Make sure you can move freely in them without getting caught in the fabric and without having them sink down.

# Getting Your Props

Once you've got your clothing figured out, there are a few more things you might need to help your practice. These items are listed in order of necessity.

YOGA MAT: This is a definite must-have. When shopping for a mat, place your hand on it to see if it slides easily. If it does, look for a different mat. You want a mat that has some stickiness or grip to it so that when you're moving through the poses or holding them for extended periods of time, your hands and feet do not slip or slide.

YOGA BLOCKS: These come in pretty standard sizes, and you really can't go wrong with your purchase. Stay away from anything that is too squishy, which might collapse if you put any weight on it; otherwise, any yoga block should work. If you're purchasing blocks, then buy two. Having the second one will make some of the poses easier to access.

YOGA STRAP: Yoga straps are pretty standard as well. They should be approximately as long as you are tall or even longer. Make sure there is a metal or plastic attachment on one end that allows you to make an adjustable loop.

BOLSTER: This is like a giant, superfirm pillow. These are great for relaxing or restorative poses. Of course, you can also just use a pillow or two to get the same effect.

BLANKET: Yoga blankets are usually made of wool and are pretty strong and durable. They have many different uses, but again, you can improvise by using any blanket you have around the house.

# Setting Up Your Space

After you have all the essentials you might need, you'll want to set up your yoga space:

1. Lay down your mat.

2. Place your props close by.

3. Keep the blocks at the front of the mat and put everything else to the side.

When you're finished practicing, roll up your mat and put it away. If your space is limited like mine, use a basket or other container to hold your mat and all your props. Keep everything together and store it conveniently so you're ready to practice again tomorrow.

Once you've got your mat laid out and you're dressed in your yoga clothes, it's time to relax.

# Relaxing

Relaxation is a key component to yoga. In fact, Patanjali says it best:

*Practicing yoga in a relaxed manner with strength creates harmony within the body.*
SUTRA 2.46, STHIRA SUKHAM ASANAM

*Sthira* means "strong and steady." *Sukham* means "comfortable and relaxed." Combine these two and you get an asana, or pose that works to create a happy body.

Here's a simple way to demonstrate the important balance between strength and relaxation:

1. Sit up straight in a comfortable position.

2. Notice which of your muscles are working and which ones are not. Your core is engaged to keep you upright, but your shoulders are relaxed.

3. Tense your shoulders and bring them toward your ears. Suddenly this becomes a very uncomfortable pose. There is no way you'd be able to hold this for any extended period of time.

4. Relax your shoulders. Now sitting there doesn't seem so hard, does it?

This is *sthira sukham asanam* in action, the balance of strength and relaxation that creates a healthy yoga practice. Another essential element is breathing.

# Breathing

Like the correlation between strength and relaxation, the body and the breath share a similar link. This connection is called *vinyasa*. If you've checked out any yoga classes in your area, you might have found that they've described them as vinyasa classes. This means they link the breath to the movement. Almost all yoga practices do this in some manner or another.

The breath is an extremely important part of the practice. It helps heat the body and also calms the mind by giving it something to focus on. However, breathing in yoga is different than the breathing you're probably doing right now as you read this.

In yoga, you breathe in and out through your nose. This is a specific method called *Ujjayi Pranayama*. It is not required, but it certainly adds to the practice. It's easy to learn—in fact, you can try it right now.

1. Place your lips together softly.

2. Breathe in through your nose.

3. Exhale out your nose.

How did that feel? Perhaps the breath you took was pretty shallow. Maybe you felt like you needed a little more air. Try it again.

1. Concentrate as you breathe through your nose.

2. Make your ribs expand by filling your lungs with air.

3. Exhale slowly.

Did that feel a little bit better? I'm guessing it did. Take it one step further.

1. Inhale slowly through your nose.

2. Let your ribs expand.

3. Keep breathing in and let your belly expand.

4. Hold it there at the top.

5. Slowly exhale.

That should've felt entirely different than the first breath you took.

Continue to breathe in this slow, deep manner. As you get more comfortable with this breathing, add a slight constriction in the back of your throat, kind of like you were trying to fog up a mirror. This will create a soft sound, like an ocean wave that should be barely audible. This breath is the *Ujjayi Pranayama.* You'll hear teachers talk about it a lot as you move through poses.

Once you learn how to breathe in this manner, you can use it to relieve stress. Stop at any point in your day, especially when you're feeling overwhelmed, and practice this breathing. After a few breaths you will be more relaxed. Try it for a minute or two and you might start to experience a stronger sense of calm.

Now imagine linking the breath with movement. You'll get another feeling that might be entirely new to you.

# Daily Poses

Before we delve deep into asana, or the practice of the physical postures, I'll teach you eight poses that you can practice daily. These are simple postures that aim to bring movement to your body, stretch out any tightness that may have developed over your day, help you relax, and keep you committed to the practice.

You can practice these poses by themselves for a short period of time or do them all together in sequence. However you choose to practice them, make sure that you pay attention to the fundamentals: Find the balance between strength and ease, and continue to breathe in a slow and conscious manner.

When it comes to poses that stretch your body, you never want to overdo it. Find that happy medium in your stretch and breathe through it. If you cannot breathe in a slow and controlled manner, you have gone too far and you should back off the stretch. This advice applies to all the poses in this book.

# Easy Pose

*Sukhasana*

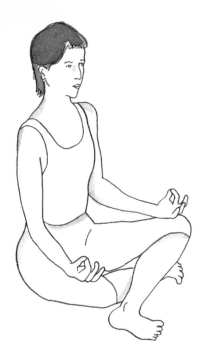

## PURPOSE

*Sukhasana* is meant to be a grounding pose where you can meditate or practice breath work.

## INSTRUCTIONS

Sit evenly on your sit bones and cross your shins in front of you. There should be space between your calves and your thighs. Once in the pose, relax your shoulders. Sit up tall. Take any extreme arch out of your back by using your abs to draw your lower ribs back into your spine.

## BREATHING

If you want to practice *ujjayi* breathing here, close your eyes and begin to breathe deeply in and out through your nose. Remember to fully fill up your lungs. Once you get the hang of it, aim for a nice, even breath so that the length of your inhale matches the length of the exhale. Try to do this for a minute or longer.

## MODIFICATIONS

While this is called Easy pose, it isn't always easy for everyone. Depending on the bone structure in your hips, this might be fairly difficult, but do not fret, because there is a modification for you. To help ease the pose, sit on something that raises your hips. This can be a bolster, blanket, or pillow or two.

# Seated Twists

*Parivrtta Sukhasana*

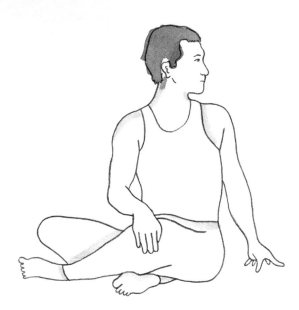

## PURPOSE

Twists are said to wring out the toxins in the body and stimulate the digestive system. When it comes to twists, you always want to twist your torso to the right first and then to the left, following the direction of the digestive path.

## INSTRUCTIONS

To begin, stay seated in Easy pose. Take your right hand and place it behind your right hip. Put your left hand on the out-side of your right knee. Inhale and sit up a little taller. Then, as you exhale use the placement of your hands as anchors to help you twist a little deeper. Hold for at least five breaths. Repeat on the other side.

## MODIFICATIONS

To modify this pose, you can place a block under your right hand so that you don't lose the upright nature in your spine. If you were seated on a blanket or a different prop in Easy pose, then continue to stay on that prop here.

# Bound Angle Pose

*Baddha Konasana*

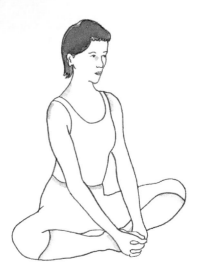

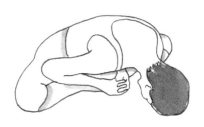

## PURPOSE

This is a great pose for opening your hips and releasing your lower back, especially if you've spent all day sitting at a desk.

## INSTRUCTIONS

From Easy pose, uncross your shins and draw the soles of your feet together. If this is a lot of stretch for the outsides of your hips, then place your hands behind you and sit up tall to support yourself. You can also sit on a blanket here as well. If your knees are far from the floor, you can also place blocks or pillows under them for support. This will help ease any strain you might feel on the outside of your legs.

## MODIFICATIONS

If your knees are fairly close to the floor and you want to deepen the stretch, bend over your legs and draw your forehead toward the soles of your feet and your torso toward the ground. Keep pressing your knees to the ground, but relax your shoulders and your neck. Hold for at least eight breaths.

# Cat/Cow

....................................

*Viralasana*

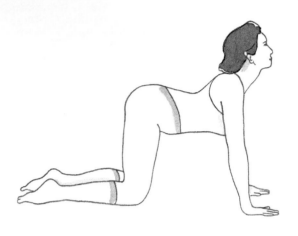

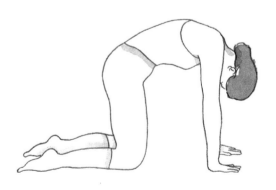

## PURPOSE

This pose helps to keep the spine supple and preps the body for moving with the breath.

## INSTRUCTIONS FOR COW

Come to your hands and knees. Place your wrists directly under your shoulders and your knees directly under your hips. As you inhale drop your belly. Let your tailbone reach toward the ceiling and keep your chest wide. This is Cow.

## INSTRUCTIONS FOR CAT

To come into Cat from Cow, exhale. Press into your hands evenly and round through your upper back. Imagine someone has his or her hand between your shoulder blades. Draw your chin to your chest and round through your spine as if you were trying to push the hand away.

Continue to move with your breath, alternating between Cat and Cow to create movement in your spine. Do this for at least five breaths.

# Low Lunge

*Anjaneyasana*

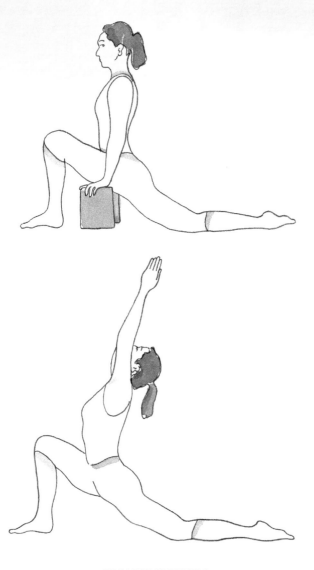

## PURPOSE

This pose is meant to open up your hip flexors, the area at the top of your thigh and front of your hip. If you spend most of your day at a desk or in your car or you are an avid runner or cyclist, then these muscles might be particularly tight. This pose will be especially good for you.

## INSTRUCTIONS

From your hands and knees, step your right foot forward so that it lands just inside your right hand. If this is a lot of stretch in your hips and groin area, then take two blocks and place them under each hand to give you some relief. To deepen the stretch, extend your arms up overhead and reach them alongside your ears. Then, allow your hips to drop toward the mat. Hold for at least eight breaths. Repeat on the other side.

## CAUTION

One note of caution here is to not let your front knee go past your ankle. If you sink your hips and notice that this is happening, step your foot forward until your knee lines up directly over your ankle.

# Sphinx

*Bhujangasana II*

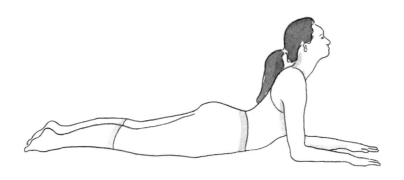

PURPOSE

This pose is considered a gentle back bend and is meant to open your chest and lengthen the front side of the body.

INSTRUCTIONS

Lie on the mat on your belly. Lift your chest off the ground and place your forearms on the mat in front of you so that your elbows are directly underneath your shoulders. Forearms should be parallel to the sides of the mat. Press your forearms down into the mat and try to drag them backward, thus making the effort to pull your chest through your arms. Your upper body should be doing all the work, and your lower body, especially your glutes, should be relaxed. Hold for at least five breaths.

# Child's Pose

*Balasana*

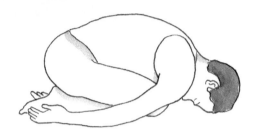

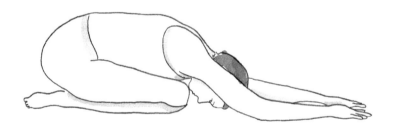

## PURPOSE

This pose is considered a resting pose. It is a great counter-pose to a back bend like Sphinx. If at any point during your practice you need a break, return to this pose.

## INSTRUCTIONS

Come to your hands and knees. Separate your knees wider than your hips and bring your big toes together. Sit back onto your heels. Walk your hands forward and allow your belly to drop between your thighs as your ribs rest on the inner thighs. Bring your forehead to the mat. Keep your arms extended forward or bring them alongside you. Hold for at least five breaths.

## MODIFICATIONS

If it is difficult to sit back on your heels, try placing a blanket or bolster on top of your calves and sit on that. This will ease any back or hip pain.

# Legs up the Wall

*Viparita Karani*

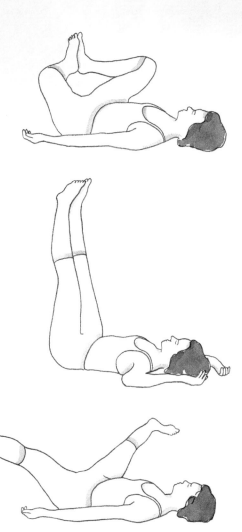

## PURPOSE

This is a great stress-relieving position. Legs up the Wall is an effective stretch for your hamstrings. You can also use it in meditation or for a final resting pose in place of Savasana.

## INSTRUCTIONS

Bring your mat to the wall. Sit next to the wall so that your right hip is pretty close to it and your legs run parallel to the wall. Lean back into your hands so that you can bend your knees and lift your legs up the wall. Lie on your back and straighten your legs up the wall to create an "L" shape with your body. Move your sit bones as close to the wall as possible. Now relax your legs, close your eyes, and breathe deeply. Hold for at least two minutes.

## VARIATION #1

To deepen the pose and stretch your inner thighs and hamstrings, allow your legs to drift apart from each other and slide down the wall, opening your legs into a "V" shape.

## VARIATION #2

To stretch your hips and lower back in this pose, bring the soles of your feet together and press your knees toward the wall. The shape of your legs should look exactly how they looked in Bound Angle pose when you were seated.

Hold each of these variations for at least five breaths.

If you're looking for a more restorative version of this pose to help you relax, try placing a blanket or a bolster under your hips while your legs are straight up the wall. Hold for at least two minutes.

## Finishing the Daily Poses

When you finish doing these eight poses, slowly make your way up to a seated position. Take a moment to check in with your body and notice any sensations you might be experiencing. Do you feel more relaxed? Less stressed? More open in your hips, back, or legs? Make a mental note of how you feel now, and then use this knowledge to motivate yourself to come back to your mat on a regular basis.

Now that you're on your way to making yoga a daily habit and you've gotten a taste of some of the poses, you're probably wondering about the others. When do you get to move? What about Down Dog, Up Dog, or that fancy pose you saw in a magazine? There's so much that the yoga poses coming up next in chapter 3 can offer; you should be excited to learn them.

CHAPTER THREE

# THE ESSENTIAL YOGA POSES

One of the greatest aspects of yoga is the idea that we can take the lessons learned on the mat off the mat. Sure, you might lose weight, tone up, or become more flexible, but the deeper things you learn on the mat, like focus and strength, can be translated into your daily life in a variety of ways. Take my story for example.

## The Power of the Poses

I have always been pretty strong. However, I have also been incredibly shy my entire life, and those two things never seemed to go together. But when I started to practice the poses, I suddenly found myself feeling strength in talking with others that I never had before. This change became apparent to me the first time I stood in front of a class full of students and taught yoga. It was then that I found my new voice, which was not the shaky one I always had since I was a shy young girl. It was the one that matched the strength of my body. Suddenly, all that I had learned on the mat spilled into my personal and professional lives. While this took years of practice to find, it is the reason I believe so strongly in the power of the poses.

This power is also why the poses tend to be the core of many yoga practices today. Practitioners use the movement of their bodies to learn the subtle and not-so-subtle lessons in life. As long as you can move your body in some form or another, even if it's just to sit comfortably and breathe, then you too can learn these. But to really grasp these lessons from the yoga poses, there are five key things to take note of as you move on your mat:

BREATH: Are you still breathing? Is it forced, or can you maintain that smooth, even *ujjayi* breath?

ALIGNMENT: Is your body properly aligned in the pose? Are your limbs in the right place?

ATTENTION: Where is your attention? Are you thinking about what you are going to have for dinner? Or, are you focused on relaxing the parts of your body that need to relax and engaging those that need to work?

GAZE: Where are you looking? Are you looking at the clock wondering if it's over yet, or are you focused on a singular point that's appropriate for the pose?

TRANSITIONS: What are you doing to get to the next pose? Are you moving mindfully with intention, or are you flopping out of the last pose quickly get to the next?

It might seem overwhelming to focus on these five things as you're learning the poses. It will get easier with practice, and soon you will reap the wide range of benefits that yoga has to offer you.

# Practicing the Poses

...............................................

The following pages describe 36 essential poses. They are meant to teach the fundamentals from which other more advanced poses can be built upon. Learning and practicing these poses prepares you to move on to other ones.

I have broken down the poses into these four sections:

1. Warm-Up

2. Standing Poses

3. Back Bends

4. Cooldown

Under each pose you will find several different categories, most of which are self-explanatory. The Preceding pose is like the warm-up to the described pose, and the Counterpose is the cooldown to the pose.

# Corpse Pose

........................................

*Savasana*

**EFFECT: A GROUNDING POSE FOR THE BEGINNING OF PRACTICE AND
A RELAXING POSE AT THE END • PROPS: BLANKET OR BOLSTER**

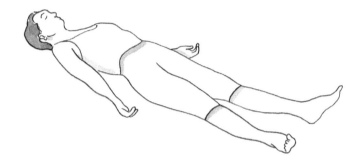

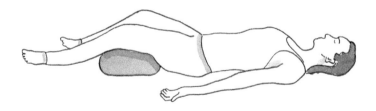

1. Lie on your back. Place your arms alongside you, palms face up. Stretch out your legs, slightly spread apart so that you're comfortable, straight in front of you on the ground.

2. Let your feet flop out to the side naturally.

3. Let your body be heavy. Relax completely.

**GAZE:** Close your eyes.

**PRECEDING POSES:** At the beginning of practice, none. At the end of practice, everything.

**COUNTERPOSES:** All poses

**PRECAUTIONS:** To modify to avoid lower back pain, you can place a blanket or bolster underneath your knees.

TIP: Relax your jaw and let your tongue fall away from the roof of your mouth to help settle deeper into the pose.

# Reclined Twists

*Jathara Parivartanasana*

**EFFECT: SPINAL WARM-UP, DETOXES BODY • PROPS: BLOCK**

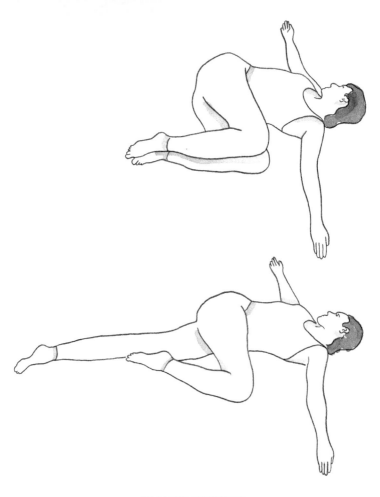

1. Lie on your back in Savasana. Bend your right knee and draw it into your chest. Keep your left leg relaxed on the ground.

2. Let your right knee fall over to the left to create a twist. Your right arm can come out to the right. Twist only as far as you can while keeping the right shoulder on the floor.

3. If it doesn't strain your neck, turn your head to the right. Repeat on the other side.

**GAZE:** Toward the ceiling or, if neck is turned, to the side

**PRECEDING POSES:** Savasana

**COUNTERPOSES:** Knees into Chest

**PRECAUTIONS:** If the twist bothers your lower back, try placing a block under the bent knee once you're in the twist. This will prevent you from placing strain on your lower back.

TIP: Another version of this twist is to do it with both knees bent.

# Down Dog

......................................

*Adho Mukha Svanasana*

**EFFECT: ENERGIZING, STRENGTHENING • PROPS: NONE**

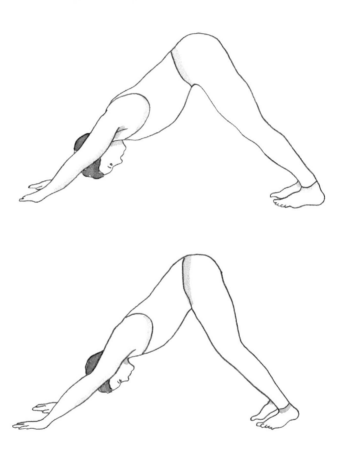

1. Come to your hands and knees. Spread your fingers wide. Make sure your hands are shoulder-distance apart and the creases of your wrists are parallel to the front of the mat.

2. Tuck your toes under and lift your hips up and back to create a "V" shape with your body.

3. Straighten your arms and roll the inner part of the elbow forward while pressing evenly through all ten fingers. Press your heels toward the mat.

4. Spin your inner thighs toward the back wall so that your heels disappear behind your second and third toes.

**GAZE:** Between your feet or at your navel

**PRECEDING POSES:** Cat/Cow, Plank, Forward Fold

**COUNTERPOSES:** Mountain pose, Extended Mountain pose

**PRECAUTIONS:** If this pose pulls too tightly on your hamstrings or bothers your lower back, bend your knees to create a sense of ease.

TIP: Don't worry if your heels do not reach the ground quite yet. One day they will get there. Keep pressing evenly into your hands. Press your heels toward the mat.

# Mountain Pose

................................................

*Tadasana*

**EFFECT: CENTERING • PROPS: NONE**

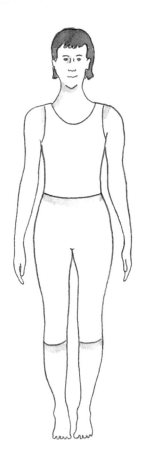

1. Stand at the front of your mat, your big toes touching and your heels slightly apart. Spread the weight evenly through all four corners of your feet.

2. Stand up tall. Spin your inner thighs toward the back wall. Engage your belly and draw your navel in. Relax your shoulders.

3. Let your arms relax alongside you. Your palms should face toward your body.

**GAZE:** Forward

**PRECEDING POSES:** Savasana

**COUNTERPOSES:** Down Dog, Forward Fold

**PRECAUTIONS:** None

TIP: This is a great time to focus inward on an intention for your practice. This can be one word or a simple mantra.

# Extended Mountain Pose

*Urdhva Hastasana*

**EFFECT: STRETCHES SHOULDERS, CENTERS • PROPS: NONE**

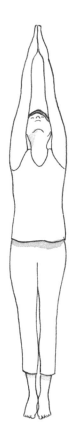
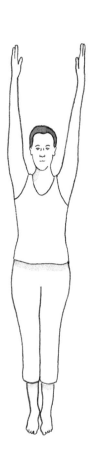

1. From Mountain pose, turn your palms to face away from you. Reach through your fingertips.

2. Keep your elbows straight and slowly circle arms up overhead. Bring your palms together to touch above you, slightly in front of your head.

3. Stand up tall. Spin your inner thighs toward the wall behind you and draw your navel in.

**GAZE:** Up toward the space between your hands

**PRECEDING POSES:** Mountain pose, Savasana

**COUNTERPOSES:** Standing Forward Fold, Down Dog

**PRECAUTIONS:** If you have any shoulder issues, keep a little bend in your elbows or do not lift your arms at all.

TIP: If your palms do not yet touch with straight arms, stop at the point where your elbows want to bend. Then, keep working on straightening through your elbows and reaching through your fingertips. This will help open your shoulders, and one day your palms will touch with straight arms.

# Standing Forward Fold

*Uttanasana*

**EFFECT: STRETCHES HAMSTRINGS, CENTERS • PROPS: NONE**

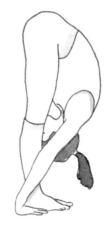

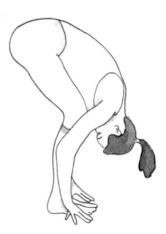

1. From Extended Mountain pose, reach your arms out to the side like a "T." Fold at your hips with a flat back.

2. Keep leading with your chest as you continue to fold. When you cannot go any further, release your hands toward the ground.

3. Relax your neck. Shift your weight from your heels to the middle of your feet.

**GAZE:** Eyes closed or toward knees

**PRECEDING POSES:** Mountain pose, Seated Forward Fold

**COUNTERPOSES:** Cobra, Sphinx

**PRECAUTIONS:** If you have any lower back issues, bend your knees.

TIP: Do not worry if your hands don't reach the ground. Keep practicing, and one day they will touch.

# Half Forward Fold

*Ardha Uttanasana*

**EFFECT: STRETCHES HAMSTRINGS, OPENS CHEST, ENERGIZES • PROPS: NONE**

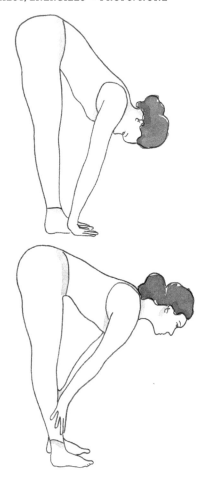

1. From Standing Forward Fold, inhale and lift your torso. Imagine doing Cow pose here. Let your belly drop and your heart lift.

2. If this is difficult to achieve with your hands on the ground, let them slide up your legs until you can open your chest and take any rounding out of your back.

3. Keep the neck and spine long.

**GAZE:** Forward to a spot in front of your mat

**PRECEDING POSES:** Standing Forward Fold, Seated Forward Fold, Cobra, Up Dog

**COUNTERPOSES:** Standing Forward Fold, Plank

**PRECAUTIONS:** If there is tightness in the hamstrings or this bothers your lower back, bend your knees.

TIP: Do not just lift your head here; work to find a tiny back bend in your upper back. Imagine pulling your spine through your chest.

# Plank

......................................

*Kumbhakasana*

**EFFECT: STRENGTHENS ENTIRE BODY
(ESPECIALLY THE CORE), ENERGIZES • PROPS: NONE**

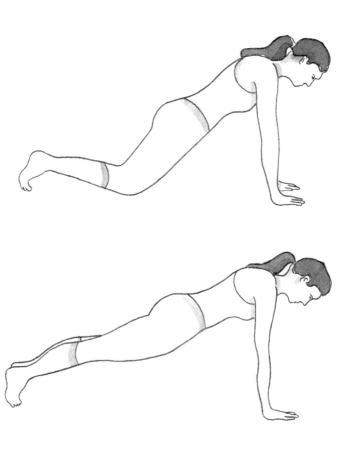

1. Come to your hands and knees. Tighten your belly muscles so that your back is flat and parallel to the ground. Extend your legs behind you. Tuck your toes under so that you end up in a push-up position.

2. Press evenly through all ten fingers and spin the inside of your elbows forward. Draw your lower belly in to avoid dropping your hips. Without moving your hips or legs, gently press your thighs toward the ceiling to engage them.

3. Press your heels back as if you're trying to step on the wall behind you. At the same time, draw your chest forward to lengthen your spine. Hold.

**GAZE:** Top of mat or tip of nose

**PRECEDING POSES:** Mountain pose

**COUNTERPOSES:** Down Dog, Cobra, Up Dog, Chaturanga

**PRECAUTIONS:** If your wrists are sensitive, you can come to your forearms and do the pose there.

TIP: If the pose is too difficult to hold and your lower belly starts to drop toward the ground, lower your knees directly below you, but do not lift your hips up.

# Four-Limbed Staff Pose

*Chaturanga*

**EFFECT: STRENGTHENS ARMS AND CORE,
BUILDS HEAT • PROPS: STRAP**

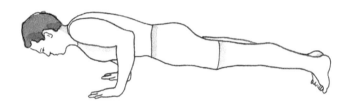

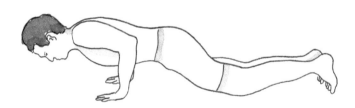

1. Start in Plank position.

2. Shift your body forward so that your shoulders are in front of your wrists.

3. Hug your elbows in toward your ribs and bend them to a 90-degree angle. Keep the rest of your body in Plank position.

**GAZE:** Front of mat

**PRECEDING POSES:**
Plank, Mountain pose

**COUNTERPOSES:** Up Dog, Cobra

**PRECAUTIONS:** If you have shoulder issues or you're still building the strength in your arms, keep your knees on the mat. Never let your shoulders drop below the height of your elbows.

TIP: To perfect your Chaturanga, try using a strap. Make a loop in the strap so that when it's flat, the edges of the loop hit the edges of your shoulders. Place the loop around your arms just above your elbows. Shift forward and bend the elbows to a 90-degree angle. You will know you've hit 90 when the strap hits your sternum and reaches across your rib cage.

# Cobra

*Bhujangasana*

**EFFECT: HEART OPENING, STRENGTHENS LOWER BACK • PROPS: NONE**

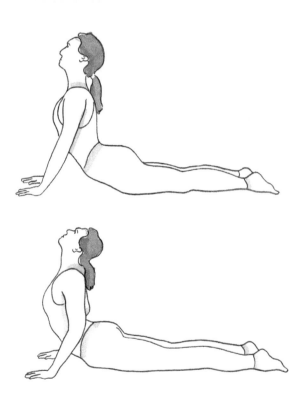

1. Lie facedown on your mat. Bend your elbows and place your hands alongside your lower ribs so that your elbows are stacked directly over your wrists.

2. Press the tops of your feet into the mat. Roll your inner thighs toward the ceiling as you hug your outer ankles in. Relax your glutes.

3. On an inhale, press into your hands and use the muscles of your lower back to lift your chest off the ground. Keep your shoulders relaxed away from your ears as you draw them back and down. Start to work your arms toward straight, but stop as soon as you feel your shoulders bunching up toward your ears.

**GAZE:** Slightly up

**PRECEDING POSES:** Plank, Chaturanga, Sphinx, Half Forward Fold

**COUNTERPOSES:** Down Dog, Standing Forward Fold

**PRECAUTIONS:** If you have lower back issues, keep your chest low and do not fully straighten your arms.

TIP: This pose can be a pretty deep back bend if you straighten your arms all the way. Only lift so high that you can keep your chest wide and your shoulders relaxed. FYI: I've been practicing for a long time, and I still don't straighten my arms all the way in this pose.

# Up Dog

*Urdhva Mukha Svanasana*

**EFFECT: HEART OPENING, STRENGTHENS
BACK AND ARMS • PROPS: NONE**

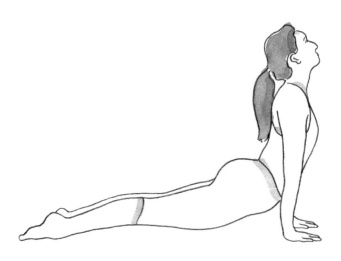

1. Lie facedown on your mat. Bend your elbows and place your hands alongside your lower ribs so that your elbows are stacked directly over your wrists.

2. Press the tops of your feet into the mat. Roll your inner thighs toward the ceiling as you hug your outer ankles in. Relax your glutes.

3. On an inhale, press into your hands to fully straighten your arms. Keep pressing the tops of your feet into the mat so that your thighs lift off the ground. Keep your shoulders relaxed away from your ears as you draw them back and down.

GAZE: Slightly up

PRECEDING POSES: Cobra, Sphinx

COUNTERPOSES: Down Dog, Standing Forward Fold

PRECAUTIONS: If you have any lower back issues, stick to Cobra with the arms bent.

TIP: Make sure to engage your legs here so that you don't let the weight of your body sink into your lower back.

# Warseguir Warrior I

*Virabhadrasana I*

**EFFECT: STRENGTHENS LEGS, FOCUSES
MIND AND BODY • PROPS: NONE**

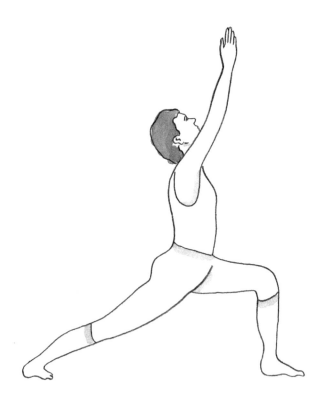

1. Stand at the front of your mat. Take a big step back with your left foot. Line up the heel of your right foot with the inside edge of your left foot. Turn your left toes slightly forward toward the left-front corner of your mat. Make sure your right toes point straight ahead.

2. Bend your right knee, working toward getting your thigh parallel to the mat. At the same time, press the pinky-side edge of your left foot into the mat and keep straightening through your left leg. Spin your left inner thigh toward the back of the room.

3. Extend your arms over-head. If elbows are straight, you can touch your palms together; otherwise, keep the arms apart. Spin your left ribs forward to square off your chest with the front of the room. Repeat on the other side.

**GAZE:** If palms are touching, gaze up toward your hands. If not, keep a soft gaze looking forward.

**PRECEDING POSES:** Low Lunge, Crescent

**COUNTERPOSES:** Down Dog, Standing Forward Fold

**PRECAUTIONS:** To protect your knees, always keep your front bent knee directly over your ankle.

TIP: It is more important to keep the back leg straight than to get the front thigh parallel to the mat. Keep rooting down through the pinky side of the back foot and straightening the back leg. If you can keep that leg straight, then you can bend deeper into the front thigh.

# Chair

......................................................

*Utkatasana*

**EFFECT: STRENGTHENS THIGHS, IMPROVES FOCUS • PROPS: NONE**

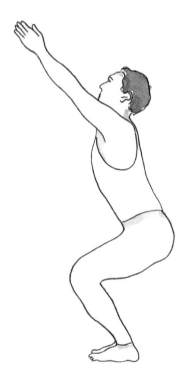

1. Stand at the top of your mat in Mountain pose.

2. Bend your knees and drop your hips as if you're sitting back in a chair.

3. Reach your arms up alongside your ears. If your elbows are straight, touch your palms together; if not, then keep your arms separated. Lift your chest as you draw your abs in.

**GAZE:** Slightly forward or up to hands if palms are touching

**PRECEDING POSES:** Mountain pose, Warrior I

**COUNTERPOSES:** Standing Forward Fold

**PRECAUTIONS:** If you have any lower back issues or are pregnant, separate your feet hip-distance apart.

TIP: Look down at your toes; if you can't see them, shift your shins backward until you can. The weight of your body should be in your heels.

# Down Dog Split

........................................

*Eka Pada Adho Mukha Svanasana*

**EFFECT: STRETCHES HAMSTRINGS AND HIPS, WORKS
ON BALANCE, CALMING • PROPS: NONE**

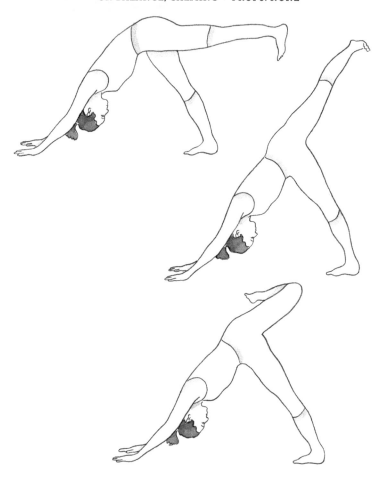

1. Start in Down Dog. Lift your right leg up toward the ceiling.

2. Continue to press evenly into all ten fingers and keep your elbows straight. Press your left heel down toward the mat.

3. To keep a square hip, keep your lifted toes facing the ground. To open your hip, turn your toes toward the side wall and bend your knee. If opening the hip, keep your shoulders square by drawing both armpits toward the ground. Repeat on the other side.

GAZE: Between feet or navel

PRECEDING POSES: Down Dog

COUNTERPOSES: Mountain pose

PRECAUTIONS: Opening the hip here may cause lower back pain; to avoid that, keep your lifted toes pointed toward the ground.

TIP: This is a great pose to use for transitions. It will help you step your foot forward when moving to standing poses.

# Crescent

......................................................

*Alanasana*

**EFFECT: STRETCHES HIP FLEXORS,
STRENGTHENS LEGS • PROPS: NONE**

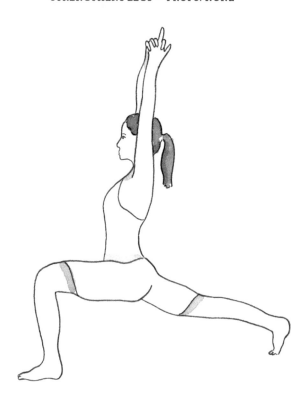

1. From Mountain pose, separate your feet hip-distance apart. Take a big step back with your left foot and bend your front knee to a 90-degree angle.

2. Draw your left hip forward to square your chest and hips off toward the front wall.

3. Extend your arms up overhead. If arms are straight, touch palms; if not, keep arms separate and reach through fingertips. Repeat on the other side.

**GAZE:** At hands if palms are touching or straight ahead if they are not

**PRECEDING POSES:** Low Lunge, Chair

**COUNTERPOSES:** Down Dog

**PRECAUTIONS:** If this pose pulls on the front of your hips, bend your back leg to ease the tension.

TIP: If it is hard to balance, try stepping your front foot toward the outside edge of the mat a few inches.

# Warrior III

......................................

*Virabhadrasana III*

**EFFECT: STRENGTHENS BACK AND LEGS, WORKS
ON BALANCE • PROPS: TWO BLOCKS**

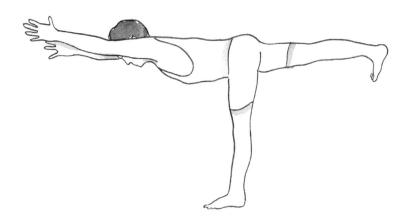

1. From Crescent pose, lean forward 45 degrees over your front thigh. Engage your belly as you reach your arms forward alongside your ears. Pause there.

2. Transfer your weight onto the front leg and lift your back leg.

3. Work to get your chest parallel to the ground. Flex through the lifted leg as if you're trying to step on the wall behind you. Repeat on the other side.

**GAZE:** Beyond the hands

**PRECEDING POSES:** Crescent, Tree

**COUNTERPOSES:** Standing Forward Fold, Mountain pose

**PRECAUTIONS:** If this pose bothers your lower back, try modifying the position of your arms by bringing hands to prayer at your heart or alongside you, reaching toward the back of the room. If it is difficult to hold your torso up, modify the pose by placing two blocks under your shoulders at their highest height. Tent your fingers on top of them and draw your chest forward.

TIP: To improve balance, press your big toe into the mat and your standing thigh toward the wall behind you. Draw the navel to the spine, but relax your shoulders.

# Standing Splits

· · · · · · · · · · · · · · · · · · · · · · · ·

*Urdhva Prasarita Eka Padasana*

**EFFECT: STRETCHES HAMSTRINGS, WORKS ON
BALANCE • PROPS: ONE OR TWO BLOCKS**

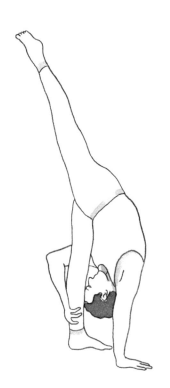
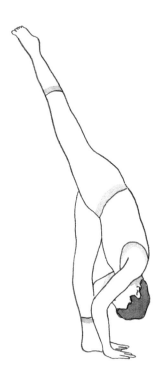

1. From Warrior III, keep your spine long as you tilt your chest forward to bring your hands down to the ground.

2. Lift your back leg up to the ceiling by lifting from your inner thigh. Keep your lifted toes pointed toward the ground to keep your hips square.

3. Draw your torso back toward your standing thigh.

**GAZE:** Down past tip of nose

**PRECEDING POSES:** Standing Forward Fold, Warrior III, Crescent

**COUNTERPOSES:** Mountain pose

**PRECAUTIONS:** If this pulls too deeply on the hamstring of the standing leg, bend your knee or use a block or two under your fingertips to get closer to the floor.

TIP: To deepen the stretch and improve balance, try placing one or both hands around your ankle.

# Warrior II

............................................

*Virabhadrasana II*

**EFFECT: STRENGTHENS LEGS, FOCUSING • PROPS: NONE**

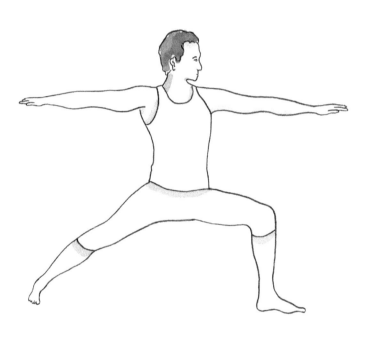

1. Stand and face the left-side wall so that your feet are wide on your mat. Turn your right toes to face forward and your left toes at a slight angle toward the left-front corner of the mat. Line up your front heel with the arch of your back foot.

2. Bend your front knee to a 90-degree angle. Aim it straight ahead over your second and third toes. Press through the pinky side of your back foot to straighten through the back leg. Keep your hips at a slight angle toward the left-front corner of your mat, but turn your chest to be parallel to the side of the mat.

3. Take your arms to shoulder height and reach them forward and back. Relax your shoulders. Keep your torso directly over your hips. Repeat on the other side.

**GAZE:** Middle finger of front hand

**PRECEDING POSES:** Warrior I, Crescent, Mountain

**COUNTERPOSES:** Down Dog, Standing Forward Fold

**PRECAUTIONS:** If the front knee juts ahead of your ankle, step your front foot forward until the knee stacks over the ankle.

TIP: Do not try to square your hips off toward the side wall; keep them at a slight angle forward so that you can bend deeper into the front thigh.

# Reverse Warrior

························································

*Viparita Virabhadrasana*

**EFFECT: STRETCHES SIDE BODY, RELAXES • PROPS: NONE**

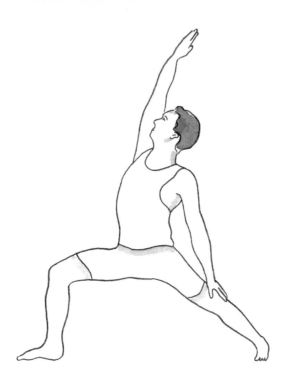

1. Start in Warrior II. Reach your front arm up toward your ear as you lean back.

2. Gently place your other hand on the top of your back thigh. Keep length in both sides of the waist.

**GAZE:** Up toward lifted hand

**PRECEDING POSES:** Warrior II

**COUNTERPOSES:**
Extended Side Angle

**PRECAUTIONS:** Make sure to engage your lower belly so as not to overarch your lower back.

TIP: Keep the front leg bent as you reach back.

# Extended Side Angle

......................................................

*Parsvakonasana*

**EFFECT: STRETCHES TORSO AND LOWER BACK,
STRENGTHENS LEGS, GROUNDING • PROPS: BLOCK**

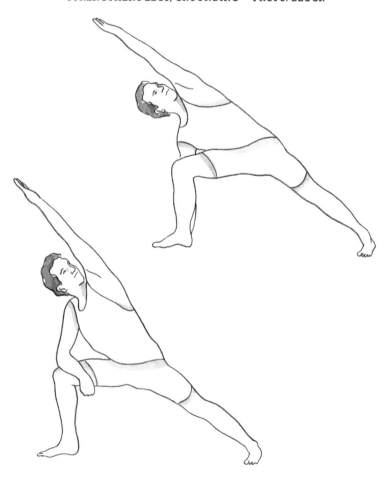

1. Start in Warrior II. Reach your front arm forward as far as possible.

2. Place your hand on the outside of the front foot. Turn your top palm toward the front of the room and reach it forward alongside your ear.

3. Roll your chest open as you hug your bottom hip underneath you.

**GAZE:** Top hand

**PRECEDING POSES:**
Warrior II, Triangle

**COUNTERPOSES:** Mountain pose, Standing Forward Fold

**PRECAUTIONS:** Beware of letting your front knee buckle in toward the middle of the mat. Draw it toward the wall behind you so that it points straight ahead.

TIP: If you cannot reach the ground with your bottom arm, try one of the following arm variations. Take your hand to the inside of your front foot. Place your hand on a block either inside or outside your foot. Put your forearm on your thigh so that it's parallel to the front of the mat.

# Triangle Pose

........................................

*Trikonasana*

**EFFECT: STRETCHES HAMSTRINGS,
STRENGTHENS CORE • PROPS: BLOCK**

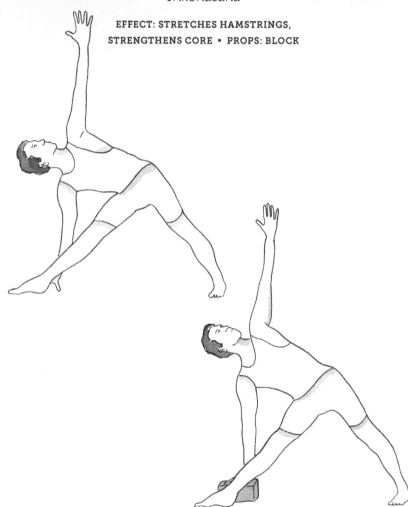

1. Start in Warrior II. Straighten your front leg.

2. Shift your hips back and reach forward as far as you can. When you can't reach any further, leave your torso where it is and let your bottom hand come down to rest either on your thigh, shin, or ankle or the ground. Reach straight up with your other hand. Stack your shoulders on top of each other.

3. Lengthen through both sides of your waist. Repeat on the other side.

**GAZE:** Top hand

**PRECEDING POSES:** Warrior II

**COUNTERPOSES:** Down Dog

**PRECAUTIONS:** If you tend to hyperextend your knees, meaning they go past straight, bend your front leg a tiny bit and press through your big toe to protect your knee joint.

TIP: To lengthen through both sides of the waist, contract the top side of your waist as if you're doing a tiny side crunch—bringing your lower ribs toward your top hip, relax the lower side waist.

# Half Moon

.........................................

*Ardha Chandrasana*

**EFFECT: WORKS ON BALANCE • PROPS: BLOCK**

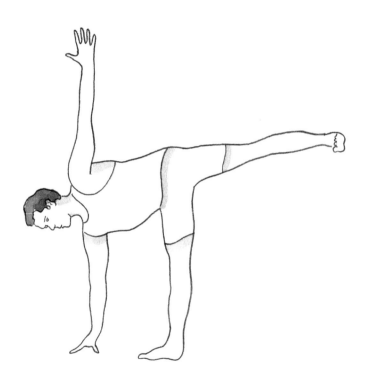

1. Start in Triangle pose. Look forward, bend your front knee, and shift your weight onto your front leg as you lift your back leg.

2. Place your bottom hand on the ground or a block and extend your other hand straight up.

3. Flex through your back heel as if you're stepping on a wall behind you. Keep your neck in line with your spine.

**GAZE:** Top hand

**PRECEDING POSES:**
Warrior II, Triangle

**COUNTERPOSES:** Standing Forward Fold, Down Dog

**PRECAUTIONS:** If it bothers your neck to gaze at your top hand, look down at your bottom hand.

TIP: The distance between your hand and your bottom foot should be the same between your armpit and the top of your hipbone. If your hand is too close to your foot, it will be difficult to balance yourself.

# Revoled Chair

.........................................

*Parivrtta Utkatasana*

**EFFECT: STRENGTHENS LEGS, DETOXES BODY,
KEEPS SPINE FLEXIBLE • PROPS: NONE**

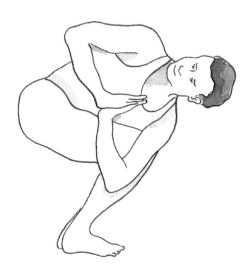

1. Start in Chair pose. Bring your hands to your heart in a prayer position.

2. Twist to the right, bringing the elbow of your left arm to the outside of your right thigh.

3. Press your right palm down into your left palm as you continue to press your left elbow on to the outside of your right thigh. Check your knees to make sure you haven't jutted one in front of the other. If you have, draw your forward knee back in line with your other knee. Repeat on the other side.

GAZE: Sideways

PRECEDING POSES: Chair pose, Seated Twists

COUNTERPOSES: Mountain pose, Standing Forward Fold

PRECAUTIONS: If you do not have enough space to get your arm to the outside of your opposite leg, separate your feet hip-distance apart and twist with open arms. Your left arm goes to the inside of your right thigh as your right arm reaches toward the ceiling and vice versa on the other side.

TIP: Use your breath to help you twist. Inhale and lengthen through your spine; exhale and twist deeper.

# Revolved Triangle

*Parivrtta Trikonasana*

**EFFECT: STRENGTHENS CORE, STRETCHES
HAMSTRINGS, DETOXES BODY • PROPS: BLOCK**

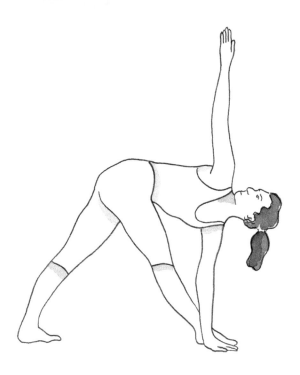

1. Start in Mountain pose. Step your left foot back about two to three feet (not as far as you would go for Warrior I). Keep your right toes pointed straight ahead, and turn your left toes at an angle to the left-front corner of your mat.

2. Square off your hips toward the front of the room. Take your right hand to your right hip and lift your left arm up alongside your ear.

3. Bend at your hips and start to fold forward. Stop when your chest is parallel to the ground.

4. Set your left fingertips on the ground or a block and twist your torso to the right. Extend your right arm to the ceiling. Repeat on the other side.

**GAZE:** Top hand

**PRECEDING POSES:**
Revolved Chair

**COUNTERPOSES:** Standing Forward Fold

**PRECAUTIONS:** If you hyperextend your knees, put a slight bend in your front leg and press through your big toe to protect your knee joint.

TIP: As you twist, keep your hips square to the ground; do not let your back hip collapse down.

# Revolved Half Moon

......................................

*Parivrtta Ardha Chandrasana*

**EFFECT: STRETCHES HAMSTRINGS, WORKS ON
BALANCE, DETOXES BODY • PROPS: BLOCK**

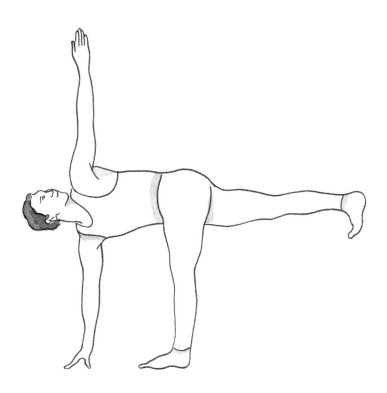

1. Start in Revolved Triangle, your right foot in front.

2. Look forward. Bend your right knee and transfer your weight to your right foot as you lift your back leg up. Place your front hand on the ground or a block as your other arm extends straight up.

3. Keep your hips square to the ground as you continue to twist your chest open to the side wall. Repeat on the other side.

**GAZE:** Top hand

**PRECEDING POSES:** Revolved Triangle, Warrior III

**COUNTERPOSES:** Standing Forward Fold, Mountain pose

**PRECAUTIONS:** If it bothers your neck to look up at your top hand, look at your bottom hand.

TIP: The tendency here is to let the hip of your lifted leg drop toward the ground as you twist. Imagine that your legs and hips are glued in one place, then twist only from your navel.

# Wide Leg Forward Fold

......................................................

*Prasarita Padottanasana*

**EFFECT: STRETCHES INNER THIGHS AND HAMSTRINGS,
CALMING • PROPS: ONE OR TWO BLOCKS**

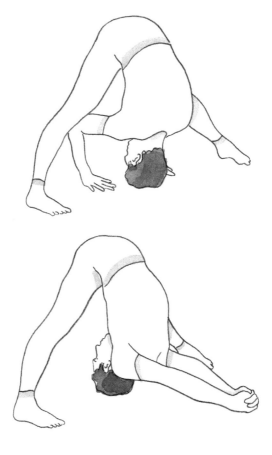

1. Stand wide on your mat, feet parallel to the sides of the mat.

2. Take your hands to your hips, inhale, and lengthen your spine; as you exhale, fold forward and bring your hands to the ground or blocks.

3. Relax your neck as you draw your inner thighs toward each other and shift your weight to the middle of your feet.

GAZE: Center of your mat or tip of your nose

PRECEDING POSES: Standing Forward Fold

COUNTERPOSES: Mountain pose, Camel, Bridge

PRECAUTIONS: If you have back issues, when coming out of the pose, bend your knees to rise back up.

TIP: For an added shoulder stretch, you can interlace your fingers behind your back and fold forward from there.

# Tree

·············································

*Vrksasana*

**EFFECT: WORKS ON BALANCE, OPENS HIPS,
IMPROVES FOCUS • PROPS: NONE**

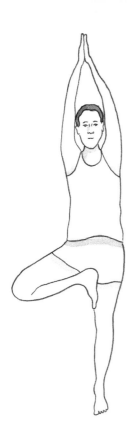 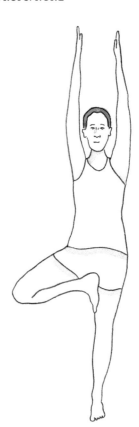

1. Start in Mountain pose. Turn your left toes out to the left and bend your knee as you bring your left foot up to the inside of your right leg.

2. Press the sole of your left foot and the inside of your right leg into each other.

3. Extend your arms overhead with straight elbows. Repeat on the other side.

**GAZE:** Up toward the ceiling

**PRECEDING POSES:** Mountain pose

**COUNTERPOSES:** Mountain pose, Standing Forward Fold

**PRECAUTIONS:** Never place the lifted foot directly on the knee joint of your standing leg. Always place it above or below the joint.

TIP: To play with your balance, try this pose with your eyes closed.

# Camel

*Ustrasana*

**EFFECT: OPENS THE CHEST, ENERGIZING • PROPS: BLOCK**

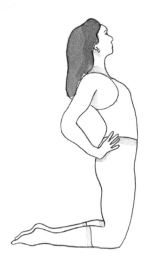

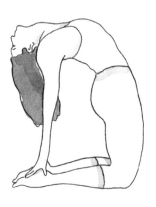

1. Kneel on your shins, toes tucked under and behind you. Place your hands on the back of your pelvis; your fingers can point up or down. Draw your elbows toward each other so they point straight back.

2. Press your thighs forward with glutes relaxed as you imagine going up and over a beach ball with your upper spine.

3. Bring your hands to your heels. Keep pressing the chest up and thighs forward.

**GAZE:** Tip of your nose

**PRECEDING POSES:** Cobra, Up Dog, Half Forward Fold

**COUNTERPOSES:** Child's pose, Seated Forward Fold

**PRECAUTIONS:** If you have any lower back issues, keep this back bend smaller by maintaining your hands on your sacrum.

TIP: If it is difficult to reach your heels, try placing a block on top of them and reach for that instead.

# Bridge

........................................

*Setu Bandha Sarvangasana*

**EFFECT: OPENS THE CHEST AND LUMBAR SPINE,
INVIGORATES • PROPS: BLOCK**

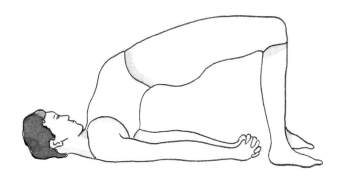

1. Lie on your back. Bend your knees. Place your feet flat on the ground, hip-distance apart and parallel to the side of the mat. Stack your knees directly over your ankles. Place your arms alongside you, palms face down.

2. When you inhale, press down into your feet to lift your hips up toward the ceiling.

3. Roll your shoulders toward each other under-neath you. Interlace your fingers. Reach your chest toward the wall behind you and tailbone to the backs of your knees.

**GAZE:** Up toward the ceiling

**PRECEDING POSES:** Cobra, Sphinx

**COUNTERPOSES:** Happy Baby, Knees into Chest

**PRECAUTIONS:** If you have lower back issues, try turning this into a restorative pose. To do so, place a block on its low or medium height underneath your sacrum, the boniest part of the back of your pelvis.

TIP: If it is difficult to clasp your hands underneath you, grab the sides of your mat and push down and forward.

# Happy Baby

......................................

*Ananda Balasana*

**EFFECT: RELEASES LOWER BACK, STRETCHES
HIPS, RELAXES • PROPS: NONE**

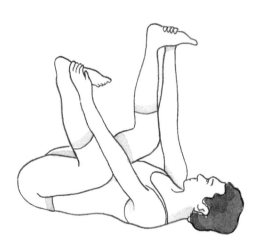

1. Lie on your back. Hug both knees into your chest.

2. Place your arms on the inside of your legs and grab onto the outsides of your feet.

3. Draw your knees toward your armpits as you keep pressing your tailbone into the mat.

**GAZE:** Up toward the ceiling

**PRECEDING POSES:** Bridge

**COUNTERPOSES:** Knees into Chest, Savasana

**PRECAUTIONS:** If it is difficult to get your hands onto your feet, try grabbing your shins or calves instead.

TIP: To deepen the stretch in the backs of your legs, try straightening your legs.

# Seated Staff

........................................

*Dandasana*

**EFFECT: PREPARES THE BODY FOR ALL SEATED
POSTURES, CALMS • PROPS: BLANKET**

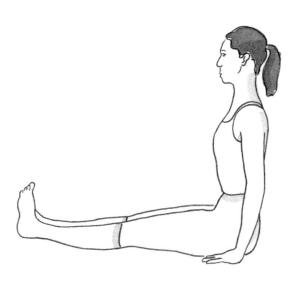

1. Sit on the mat with your legs stretched out in front of you.

2. Take your arms alongside you, palms face down. Sit up tall.

3. Flex your feet, drawing your toes back toward your body.

**GAZE:** Straight ahead

**PRECEDING POSES:**
Mountain pose

**COUNTERPOSES:** Savasana

**PRECAUTIONS:** If you have a deep round in your back, try sitting up against a wall to help hold your spine upright.

TIP: If your hamstrings are tight and it is difficult to sit up with a straight spine, then place a blanket underneath your sit bones.

# Seated Forward Fold

........................................

*Paschimottanasana*

**EFFECT: STRETCHES HAMSTRINGS,
CALMS • PROPS: BLOCK AND BLANKET**

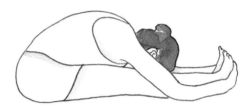

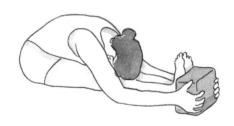

1. Start in Seated Staff pose. Inhale and reach your arms up alongside your ears.

2. On an exhale, start to reach forward. Lead with your chest and do not round your back.

3. When you can't reach any further, let your hands come down either to the ground or the outside of your legs or clasp your feet.

**GAZE:** Toes

**PRECEDING POSES:** Standing Forward Fold, Seated Staff pose

**COUNTERPOSES:** Savasana

**PRECAUTIONS:** If your hamstrings are tight, try sitting on a blanket.

TIP: If you are super flexible and can easily reach your toes, try placing a block against the bottoms of your feet. Then reach for the top of the block to bring you deeper into the pose.

# Half Lord of the Fishes

......................

*Ardha Matsyendrasana*

**EFFECT: STRETCHES SPINE, PROMOTES
HEALTHY DIGESTION • PROPS: BLOCK**

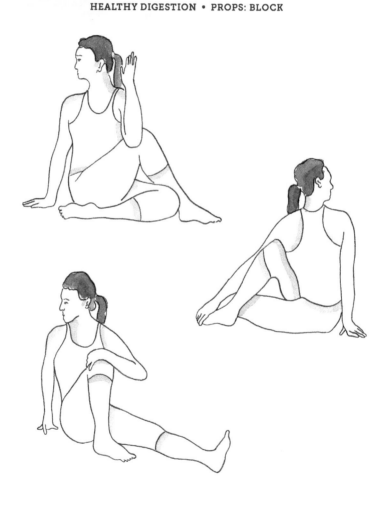

1. Start in Seated Staff pose. Bend your right knee and step your foot over your left thigh and set it on the outside of your left leg.

2. Bend your left leg and bring your heel toward your right sit bone. Sit up tall.

3. Place your right hand behind you and lift your left hand up to the ceiling. As you exhale, twist to the right and bring your left elbow to the outside of your right knee. Repeat on the other side.

**GAZE:** Over your back shoulder

**PRECEDING POSES:** Seated Twists, Revolved Chair

**COUNTERPOSES:** Seated Forward Fold

**PRECAUTIONS:** When you bend the second leg underneath you, if you cannot keep both sit bones on the ground, then unbend the leg and do this pose with the bottom leg straight.

TIP: If your back hand does not reach the floor, place a block underneath it. Use your breath to twist deeper. Inhale, sit up tall, and exhale as you twist further.

# Seated Wide Leg Forward Fold

·········································

*Upavista Konasana*

**EFFECT: STRETCHES HAMSTRINGS AND INNER
THIGHS, CALMS • PROPS: BLANKET, BOLSTER**

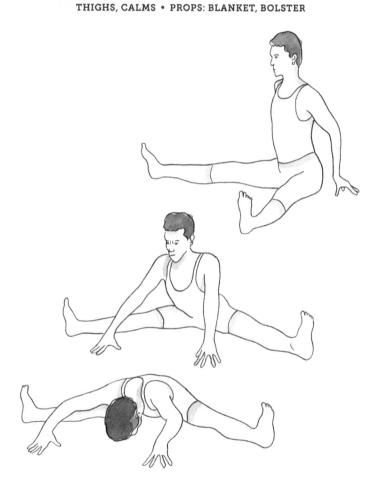

1. Start in Seated Staff pose. Bring your legs apart to form a wide "V" shape.

2. Flex your feet and straighten through your legs. Your kneecaps and toes should face the ceiling.

3. Place your hands behind you and sit up tall. Keep length in your spine as you fold forward, walking your hands with you.

**GAZE:** Forward

**PRECEDING POSES:** Seated Forward Fold, Wide Leg Forward Fold

**COUNTERPOSES:** Bound Angle pose

**PRECAUTIONS:** If it is difficult to sit up straight, place a blanket under your hips. Do not fold forward if this causes your back to round.

TIP: To turn this into a restorative pose, place the bolster in front of you, fold forward, and lay your chest on top of it.

# Reclined Pigeon

......................................

*Supta Kapotasana*

**EFFECT: STRETCHES HIPS, CALMS • PROPS: NONE**

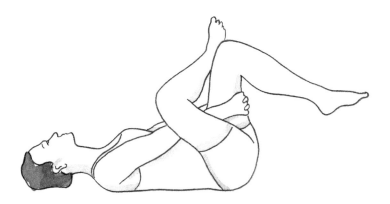

1. Lie on your back. Bend your knees and place your feet on the mat.

2. Place your right ankle just above your left knee.

3. Slide your right hand through the space between your legs and grab behind your left thigh with both hands. Draw your left thigh toward your chest. Flex your right foot and press your knee toward the wall in front of you. Repeat on the other side.

**GAZE:** Up toward the ceiling or eyes closed

**PRECEDING POSES:** Bound Angle, Seated Wide Leg Forward Fold

**COUNTERPOSES:** Knees into Chest, Reclining Hand-to-Toe pose

**PRECAUTIONS:** If your hips are extremely tight, you can leave your bottom foot on the ground and keep your arms relaxed alongside you.

TIP: To deepen the stretch, try grabbing the top of your shin instead of the back of your thigh. This will allow you to draw the top leg closer to your chest.

# Reclining Hand-to-Toe Pose

*Supta Padangusthasana*

**EFFECT: STRETCHES HAMSTRINGS, INNER THIGHS, IT (ILIOTIBIAL)
BAND, AND LOWER BACK, CALMS • PROPS: STRAP**

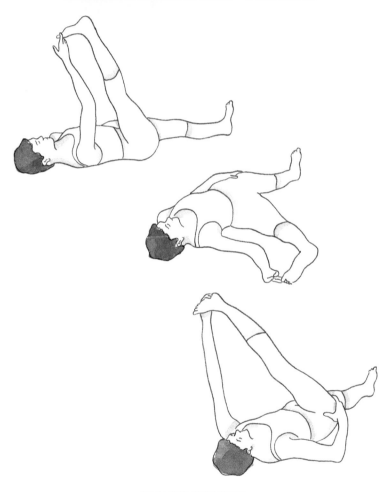

1. Lie down on your back. Lift your right leg up to the ceiling and grab your big toe with your index and middle fingers. Straighten your leg and relax your shoulders. Your left leg should remain extended on the ground. Hold for five breaths.

2. Allow your right leg to fall over to the right, but go only so far as you can while keeping your left hip and left sit bone on the mat. Hold for five breaths.

3. Come back through the center. Grab your right foot with your left hand and allow your leg to go to the left for a stretch and a twist. It is okay to let your right sit bone lift here. Hold for five breaths. Repeat on the other side.

**GAZE:** Big toe

**PRECEDING POSES:** Seated Forward Fold

**COUNTERPOSES:** Bridge with a block under your sacrum, Savasana

**PRECAUTIONS:** Most people have difficulty reaching their feet with their hands. You can place a strap around the sole of your foot and place the two sides of the strap into your hands. Move as directed.

TIP: As you take your leg across your body, try going only a few inches at first. This might deepen the stretch along the outside of the leg. This is especially great for runners.

# Corpse Pose

........................................

*Savasana*

**EFFECT: A GROUNDING POSE FOR THE BEGINNING OF PRACTICE AND
A RELAXING POSE AT THE END • PROPS: BLANKET OR BOLSTER**

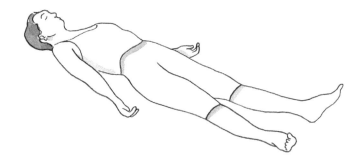

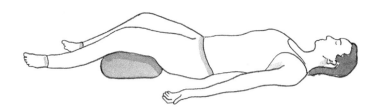

We've already touched on this pose once before. However, because this is the pose that you'll end every practice with, it seems appropriate to address how to come out of the pose here.

1. From Savasana, start to deepen your breath. Wiggle your fingers and your toes and reach up overhead to stretch through your body.

2. Draw your knees into your chest and roll onto your right side.

3. Gently press your way up into a comfortable seated position.

4. Bring your hands to prayer and gently bow your head to your hands, taking a moment to acknowledge all the work you did.

**GAZE:** Close your eyes.

**PRECEDING POSES:** At the end of practice, everything.

**COUNTERPOSES:** All poses

**PRECAUTIONS:** To modify to avoid lower back pain, you can place a blanket or bolster underneath your knees.

TIP: This is the point of practice where you would say *namaste*, which means "The divine light in me salutes the divine light in you."

CHAPTER FOUR

# SEQUENCES

Sequences are combinations of the poses put together in order to create a specific outcome or effect. You could practice a sequence with a lot of core and leg work that could be used as a workout. You might mix the daily poses with a few cooldown poses to create a calming effect. Or, you could get more specific with your needs and create a sequence to stretch tight hips or relieve back pain.

There are endless possibilities for creating sequences. However, there are three essential components that you need to know:

VINYASA: While *vinyasa* means "linking the breath to movement," it also describes a set of poses that help you move from one to another. In classes you will often hear teachers say, "Take a Vinyasa," which is shorthand for several different poses that will be described below.

**SUN SALUTATION A:** This is one of the most traditional sequences. It can be done on its own or in combination with other poses. If done on its own, it is a great way to start or end the day. If done in combination with other poses, it is used as a way to warm up the body in preparation for a longer sequence.

**SUN SALUTATION B:** Like Sun Salutation A, Sun Salutation B is a traditional sequence. It can be done alone or in combination with Sun Salutation A or a variety of poses to create a longer sequence.

You will find detailed descriptions of these three components in the next few sections. Once you learn how you move the body in these short sequences, you can reference them to help you understand how to move in all the other ones.

# Vinyasa

This short little sequence is a way to get from standing poses back to Down Dog, which is where most of the poses in a sequence will start and end. There are two versions of a Vinyasa: Version One and Version Two.

# Vinyasa

.........................................

## Version One—modified

*Do this version if it is difficult to lower through Chaturanga without letting your belly drop or if you have any lower back issues.*

**PLANK**

.....................................................

**CHATURANGA WITH KNEES ON THE GROUND**

.....................................................

**COBRA**

.....................................................

**DOWN DOG**

1. Come to Plank from whatever pose you were in previously.

2. Lower your knees to the mat.

3. Exhale and shift your shoulders forward. Bend your elbows to a 90-degree angle for Chaturanga.

4. Lower your body to the mat.

5. Inhale and lift your chest to come into Cobra.

6. On an exhale, lower your chest toward the mat. Bend your knees and press your hips back as if you were coming into Child's pose.

7. Tuck your toes under. Press into your hands and lift your hips up and back to come into Down Dog.

# Vinyasa

......................................

*Version Two*

*Choose this version if you can keep your body in Plank as you lower through Chaturanga.*

**PLANK**

**CHATURANGA**

**UP DOG**

**DOWN DOG**

1. Come to Plank from whatever pose you were in previously.

2. Exhale and shift your shoulders forward. Bend your elbows to a 90-degree angle for Chaturanga.

3. Inhale and straighten your arms. Open your chest and uncurl your toes to come into Up Dog.

4. Exhale, curl your toes under, and lift your hips up and back to come to Down Dog.

# Sun Salutation A
# (Sun Salute A)

*Surya Namaskar A*

*This is a great warm-up sequence that can be used within a larger sequence or repeated on its own for a shorter practice to wake up the body. You will also find variations of Sun Salute A in almost all sequences.*

MOUNTAIN POSE

EXTENDED MOUNTAIN POSE

STANDING FORWARD FOLD

HALF FORWARD FOLD

VINYASA—(PLANK, CHATURANGA, COBRA OR UP DOG, DOWN DOG)

HALF FORWARD FOLD

STANDING FORWARD FOLD

EXTENDED MOUNTAIN POSE

MOUNTAIN POSE

1. From Mountain pose, inhale and circle your arms overhead for Extended Mountain pose.

2. Exhale and fold forward to come into Standing Forward Fold.

3. Inhale and lift your chest for Half Forward Fold.

4. Exhale and step back to Plank to take a Vinyasa: Lower through Chaturanga. Inhale and lift your chest for Cobra or Up Dog. Exhale back to Down Dog.

5. Hold Down Dog for five breaths. ❯

6. At the end of your fifth exhale, look forward and gently step your feet together between your hands.

7. Inhale. Lift your torso for Half Forward fold.

8. Exhale. Lower your torso for Standing Forward Fold.

9. Inhale. Circle your arms out to the side as you rise up to stand in Extended Mountain pose.

10. Exhale. Bring your arms alongside you for Mountain pose.

11. Repeat as many times as desired.

# Sun Salutation B
# (Sun Salute B)

*Surya Namaskar B*

*Like Sun Salute A, Sun Salute B is a great way to warm up the body. Sun Salute B, however, takes the practice a little further by incorporating the major muscles of the legs, thus making it a bit more athletic and invigorating.*

MOUNTAIN POSE

CHAIR

STANDING FORWARD FOLD

HALF FORWARD FOLD

VINYASA—(PLANK, CHATURANGA, COBRA OR UP DOG, DOWN DOG)

WARRIOR I ON RIGHT SIDE

VINYASA—(PLANK, CHATURANGA, COBRA OR UP DOG, DOWN DOG)

WARRIOR I ON LEFT SIDE

VINYASA—(PLANK, CHATURANGA, COBRA OR UP DOG, DOWN DOG)

HALF FORWARD FOLD

STANDING FORWARD FOLD

CHAIR

EXTENDED MOUNTAIN POSE

MOUNTAIN POSE

1. From Mountain pose, inhale and circle your arms overhead to sit back into Chair.

2. Exhale, fold forward, and then straighten your legs to come into Standing Forward Fold.

3. Inhale and lift your chest for Half Forward Fold.

4. Exhale and step back to Plank to move through a Vinyasa: Lower through Chaturanga. On an inhale, lift your chest for Cobra or Up Dog. Exhale back to Down Dog. ❯

*Sun Salutation B, continued*

5. From Down Dog, step your right foot forward on the inside of your right wrist and lower your back heel down. On an inhale, rise up to Warrior I.

6. On an exhale, bring your hands to the mat and step back to Plank to move through a Vinyasa.

7. Repeat Warrior I on the left side. Then take a Vinyasa back to Down Dog.

8. Hold Down Dog for five breaths.

9. At the end of your fifth exhale, look forward and gently step your feet together between your hands.

10. As you inhale, lift your torso for Half Forward Fold.

11. On an exhale, lower your torso for Standing Forward Fold.

12. On an inhale, circle your arms up alongside your ears as you bend your knees and drop your hips to come into Chair.

13. Exhale, stand up, and bring your arms alongside you for Mountain pose.

14. Repeat as many times as desired.

# Beginner Sequences

This section contains 10 solid sequences that are great for beginners: Calming, Hip Opening, Heart Opening, Back Pain Relief, Energizing, Detoxing, Strong Legs, Balancing, Short & Sweet, and The Ultimate Sequence. They vary in length and purpose, but all work to give you the benefits of yoga practice.

Here are a few things to note while practicing the sequences:

+ To move from pose to pose, you will take a Vinyasa between each pose. One thing to note here is that while taking a Vinyasa is a great way to get from the standing poses back to Down Dog, it can be pretty challenging. Feel free to skip Vinyasas at any point during the practice. Instead of moving through a Vinyasa to return to Down Dog, all you have to do is step back to Plank and lift your hips to Down Dog.

+ Make sure that you repeat any pose that is one-sided on the other side.

+ At the end of your practice, try to stay in Savasana or the final resting pose for at least five minutes.

# Calming

*This sequence is meant to help you unwind after a stressful day. The focus in this sequence should be on the breath.*

*Hold each pose for eight breaths, except for the poses in Sun Salute A, where you'll breathe one breath per movement. The entire sequence should take 20 to 30 minutes; however, you can extend the sequence by holding the poses longer.*

1. Easy pose

2. Seated Twists

3. Cat/Cow (four or five cycles)

4. Down Dog

5. Low Lunge

6. Sun Salute A (twice)

7. Step to the front of the mat from Down Dog

8. Wide Leg Forward Fold

9. Triangle

10. Sun Salute A to end in Down Dog

11. Child's pose

12. Happy Baby

13. Reclined Hand-to-Toe pose

14. Reclined Twists

15. Savasana

# Hip Opening

...........................................

*This sequence is meant to work on releasing any tension or tightness you might feel in your hips. It is said that people hold emotions in their hips. As you practice this sequence, embrace the release and let go of anything you are holding on to, both physically and emotionally.*

*Except for the Sun Salutes and where otherwise indicated, hold each pose for five breaths. The sequence should take about 45 minutes.*

1. Savasana

2. Happy Baby (hold for 10 breaths)

3. Reclined Pigeon (hold for 10 breaths on each side)

4. Low Lunge

5. Down Dog

6. Vinyasa

7. Sun Salute A (twice)

8. Down Dog Split with square hip

9. Crescent

10. Vinyasa (repeat poses 8 to 10 for your other side)

11. Sun Salute B

12. Down Dog Split with open hip

13. Warrior II

14. Reverse Warrior

15. Extended Side Angle

16. Vinyasa (repeat poses 12 to 16 for your other side) ❱

*Hip Opening, continued*

17. Child's pose

18. Half Lord of the Fishes

19. Seated Wide Leg
Forward Fold

20. Bound Angle pose
(hold for 10 breaths)

21. Reclined Pigeon (hold
for 10 breaths on each side)

22. Reclined Twists

23. Savasana

# Heart Opening

........................................

*A heart-opening sequence will stretch and open your chest and shoulders. This helps to counteract any sitting or slouching you may do during the day. Practicing heart-opening poses causes you to feel more open and receptive to love and the goodness around you.*

*Except for the Sun Salutes and where otherwise indicated, hold each pose for five breaths. The sequence should take about 45 minutes.*

1. Easy pose

2. Cat/Cow

3. Plank

4. Chaturanga (lower to your belly)

5. Sphinx (three times)

6. Child's pose

7. Down Dog

8. Low Lunge

9. Vinyasa (repeat poses 8 and 9 for your other side)

10. Sun Salute A (twice)

11. Crescent (with arms extended by ears, try leaning upper torso back to create a slight back bend)

12. Vinyasa (repeat poses 11 and 12 for your other side)

13. Crescent (interlace your fingers behind your back)

14. Remain in Crescent pose (with your fingers still interlaced behind your back, lean forward over your front thigh at a 45-degree angle) ❱

**15.** Warrior III (keep fingers interlaced behind your back)

**16.** Standing Splits

**17.** Standing Forward Fold

**18.** Half Forward Fold

**19.** Vinyasa (repeat poses 13 to 19 for your other side)

**20.** Camel (three times)

**21.** Child's pose

**22.** Bridge

**23.** Happy Baby

**24.** Reclined Pigeon (hold for 10 breaths on each side)

**25.** Reclined Hand-to-Toe

**26.** Reclined Twists

**27.** Savasana

# Back Pain Relief

*This sequence is meant to ease everyday aches and pains in the back. If you have a more serious spinal injury, I suggest checking with your doctor to see what poses are right for you.*

*Hold each pose for eight breaths, except where noted. The sequence should take 15 to 20 minutes.*

1. Savasana

2. Reclined Twists (place a block under your bent knee to support your lower back)

3. Reclined Pigeon (hold for two minutes on each side)

4. Reclining Hand-to-Toe

5. Happy Baby

6. Reclined Twists with both knees together

7. Savasana

# Energizing

*This sequence is a little bit more challenging than the preceding ones, but like any good workout, it will leave you feeling energized and ready for the day.*

*Except for the Sun Salutes, hold each pose for five breaths. This sequence takes about an hour to complete.*

1. Savasana

2. Reclined Twists

3. Cat/Cow

4. Plank (try to hold for one minute before taking a Vinyasa or coming to Down Dog)

5. Sun Salute A (twice)

6. Sun Salute B (twice)

7. Warrior II

8. Reverse Warrior

9. Extended Side Angle

10. Warrior II

11. Triangle

12. Half Moon

13. Standing Forward Fold

14. Half Forward Fold

15. Vinyasa (repeat poses 7 to 15 for your other side)

16. Child's pose

17. Bridge (three times)

18. Happy Baby

19. Seated Staff

20. Seated Forward Fold

21. Bound Angle

22. Reclined Twists

23. Savasana

# Detoxing

*It is said that twists are great for wringing out toxins in the body. Whether these toxins are in food and drinks or simply part of negative thought patterns, this sequence focuses on winding and unwinding the body to let go of all that is unneeded.*

*Except for the Sun Salutes, hold each pose for five breaths. This sequence will take about an hour.*

1. Savasana

2. Reclined Twists

3. Down Dog

4. Sun Salute A (twice)

5. Sun Salute B (twice— during the last Chair, twist to each side for Revolved Chair)

6. Warrior II

7. Triangle

8. Vinyasa (repeat poses 6 to 8 for your other side)

9. Revolved Triangle

10. Revolved Half Moon

11. Standing Forward Fold

12. Half Forward Fold

13. Vinyasa (repeat poses 13 to 17 for your other side)

14. Child's pose

15. Bridge (three times)

16. Happy Baby

17. Seated Staff

18. Seated Forward Fold

19. Half Lord of the Fishes

20. Bound Angle

21. Happy Baby

22. Reclined Twists with both knees together

23. Savasana

# Strong Legs

*This sequence can be a bit more challenging than the preceding ones, as it will engage many of the major muscle groups of the legs. Remember, you can always skip Vinyasas or take Child's pose if it ever becomes too much.*

*Except for the Sun Salutes or where noted, hold all poses for five breaths. This sequence will take about an hour and fifteen minutes.*

1. Savasana
2. Reclined Twists
3. Plank
4. Down Dog
5. Sun Salute A (twice)
6. Sun Salute B (twice)
7. Warrior I
8. Warrior II
9. Reverse Warrior
10. Extended Side Angle
11. Vinyasa (repeat poses 7 to 11 for your other side)
12. Warrior I
13. Warrior II
14. Triangle
15. Vinyasa (repeat poses 12–15 for your other side)
16. Chair
17. Revolved Chair (twist to both sides here)
18. Vinyasa
19. Down Dog Split with a square hip
20. Crescent
21. Warrior III
22. Standing Splits with a square hip

23. Standing Forward Fold

24. Half Forward Fold

25. Vinyasa (repeat poses 19 to 25 for your other side)

26. Bridge (three times)

27. Happy Baby

28. Reclined Pigeon

29. Reclining Hand-to-Toe

30. Reclined Twists

31. Savasana

# Balancing

........................................

*By working on physical balance in this sequence, you will be working not only on engaging your core but also on learning the lessons of balancing in life.*

*Hold all poses for five breaths, except for the Sun Salutes. This is about a 45-minute practice.*

1. Easy pose

2. Seated Twists

3. Sun Salute A (twice)

4. Sun Salute B

5. Warrior II

6. Triangle

7. Half Moon

8. Standing Forward Fold

9. Half Forward Fold

10. Vinyasa (repeat poses 5 to 10 for other side)

11. Crescent

12. Warrior III

13. Revolved Half Moon

14. Standing Forward Fold

15. Half Forward Fold

16. Vinyasa (repeat poses 11 to 16 for your other side)

17. Tree

18. Camel (three times)

19. Child's

20. Seated Staff

21. Seated Forward Fold

22. Half Lord of the Fishes

23. Happy Baby

24. Reclined Pigeon

25. Reclined Twists

26. Savasana

# Short & Sweet

........................................

*Short on time? This sequence is for you. With just a few key poses, this sequence will leave you feeling refreshed and ready for the day.*

*Except for the Sun Salutes, hold each pose for five breaths—unless you're really short on time, then feel free to hold for shorter periods. This sequence should take 10 to 15 minutes.*

1. Easy pose

2. Seated Twists

3. Plank

4. Down Dog

5. Low Lunge

6. Sun Salute A

7. Sun Salute B

8. Revolved Chair

9. Seated Wide Leg Forward Fold

10. Bound Angle

11. Half Lord of the Fishes

12. Easy pose or Savasana

# The Ultimate Sequence

*I call this the ultimate sequence because it combines everything you know into one sequence. Essentially it is the entire set of poses from chapter 3 done in order with the added Vinyasas to help you move from pose to pose. This sequence will be incredibly challenging. Attempt to do this sequence once you have been practicing for a while.*

*Except for the Sun Salutes, hold each pose for five breaths. This sequence will take about an hour and a half.*

1. Savasana

2. Reclined Twists

3. Sun Salute A

4. Sun Salute B

5. Crescent

6. Warrior Three

7. Standing Splits

8. Standing Forward Fold

9. Half Forward Fold

10. Vinyasa (repeat poses 5 to 10 for your other side)

11. Warrior II

12. Reverse Warrior

13. Extended Side Angle

14. Vinyasa (repeat poses 11 to 14 for your other side)

15. Warrior II

16. Triangle

17. Half Moon

18. Standing Forward Fold

19. Half Forward Fold

20. Vinyasa (repeat poses 15 to 20 for your other side)

21. Chair

22. Revolved Chair (twist to both sides)

23. Mountain

24. Revolved Triangle

25. Revolved Half Moon

26. Standing Forward Fold

27. Half Forward Fold

28. Vinyasa (repeat poses 23 to 28 for your other side)

29. Mountain

30. Wide Leg Forward Fold

31. Tree

32. Camel

33. Bridge (three times)

34. Happy Baby

35. Seated Staff

36. Seated Forward Fold

37. Half Lord of the Fishes

38. Bound Angle

39. Reclined Pigeon (hold for eight breaths on each side)

40. Reclined Hand-to-Toe

41. Reclined Twists

42. Savasana

While the sequences listed in this chapter can be practiced endlessly, you might find yourself wanting more, which is why I'd like to teach you how to create a sequence of your own.

# Building Your Own Sequence

Creating a sequence on your own might seem intimidating at first. However, the more you practice, the more you'll be able to listen to your body and create a sequence that's appropriate for you in the moment. As you move, you'll understand what feels good and what feels awkward. For now, I've put together a few guidelines to help you get started.

**CREATE A BEGINNING, A MIDDLE, AND AN END TO YOUR SEQUENCE.** Make sure that your sequence contains at least one element from each of the following categories:

1. Warm up

2. Sun Salutations

3. Standing poses

4. Back bends

5. Cool down

6. Savasana

**MOVE THE BODY AND ITS JOINTS IN ALL DIRECTIONS.** With every sequence you create, you want to make sure that your body gets to move in a well-rounded manner.

**CHOOSE THE ORDER OF YOUR POSES WISELY.** As you may have noticed in the previous chapter, every pose had preceding and counterposes listed next to it. This is meant to help practitioners understand why we put the poses in a certain order. With every pose you practice, you want to make sure that you warm up the correct body parts and then cool down or counteract the physical effects of the pose. For example, after a back bend like Bridge, draw your knees into your chest or do Happy Baby. That way, the spine goes in the opposite direction from what it was just in when you were in Bridge.

**FOCUS ON A THEME.** Try this if you're not sure where to start in making a sequence. This can be as easy as practicing breathing, or it can be as challenging as focusing on a certain area of the body, like the legs or hips.

Above all else, have fun with your practice and listen to your body. If something doesn't feel right, then don't do it.

CHAPTER FIVE

# NUTRITION

Good nutrition complements yoga practice in a variety of ways. If I eat a big salad for lunch and follow it with a glass of water, I feel energized. But if I eat a bowl of mac and cheese and a slice of garlic bread and wash it down with a soda, I may feel happy in the moment, because I love mac and cheese, but I'll soon feel lethargic and heavy.

If you commit to a daily yoga practice in some form or another, the latter type of eating starts to affect more than just energy. Imagine trying to sit in Easy pose and breathing consciously when your stomach is full of cheese and butter. That doesn't leave much room for the lungs to expand, and it will definitely give you a whole other feeling than the calming one you're trying to achieve. How would it feel in Warrior II or Chair if you were lethargic or too full with processed foods to breathe consciously? You probably wouldn't enjoy yoga that much, and you might shy away from it. It's a matter of making good choices.

# Making Better Choices

Here's the good news. The more you commit to yoga, the better you'll feel about yourself, regardless of your current size or health. And when you feel good about your body, you tend to make better choices.

Good nutrition is all about good choices that come from sound information. If you're worried about the way you eat, consult your doctor or a nutritionist to find out specific ways to improve your eating habits.

*Ahimsa*, doing no harm, comes into play here. When you're making choices about food, ask yourself, "Is this going to hurt me or is it going to promote health?" Most of the time if you ask this single question, you'll make the correct choice. But of course you're human. So, when you have a slice of cake or eat that pint of ice cream, don't beat yourself up about it, because that does no good. Remember, you want to "do no harm." Punishing yourself for eating poorly every now and then is not very nice to your body or your mind.

# Improving Eating Habits

In general you should try to eat in a slow and mindful manner. This can mean turning off the TV while you eat or walking away from your computer. Do your best to eat whole organic foods and meats that are raised ethically. Try eating local and supporting your neighborhood farmers' market. What works for your neighbor or that model in some ad in a magazine may not work for you. It's useful then to practice *satya*, or truthfulness.

Remember yoga is practice, not perfection, and this applies to eating as well. You do not need to eat in one specific way in order to be a "good yogi." Simply eat in a manner that makes you the healthiest version of yourself.

# Styles of Eating

I wholeheartedly believe that you can find a mindful manner of eating that works for you and your body that will also complement your yoga practice. It's also true that there are various cooking styles that have been associated with the yoga lifestyle. This section contains a small sampling of different cooking styles that you can follow for one meal or every one. They are meant to be informative so that you can make the choices that do the least harm to you.

The five styles of eating that will be discussed:

1. Vegetarian

2. Vegan

3. Ayurvedic

4. Raw food

5. Acid alkaline

## Vegetarian

The vegetarian way of eating can be summed up into two words: no animals. Vegetarians refrain from eating meat, fish, and poultry. There are three types of vegetarians:

OVO: Refrains from consuming meat, fish, poultry, and milk but will eat eggs.

LACTO: Refrains from eating meat, fish, poultry, and eggs but will consume milk.

OVO-LACTO: Refrains from eating meat, fish, and poultry but will consume eggs and milk.

Beyond the aforementioned types of vegetarians, there are some people who will identify as vegetarian but will be semi-vegetarian—eating fish and poultry, but no red meat—and others will take a pescatarian approach—eating fish.

People become vegetarians for many reasons. In the yoga lifestyle, one of the main reasons is the principle of *ahimsa*. These vegetarians refrain from eating meat because they do not believe in killing animals for food. However, others become vegetarian for health or ecological reasons, sheer economics, or the fact that they simply dislike meat.

Oftentimes people become vegetarian for one reason and adopt another reason later on down the line. While there can be many benefits to eating a vegetarian or semi-vegetarian diet, there are some downfalls as well. When eating a vegetarian diet, you want to include whole, organic, and minimally processed foods, and you want to go easy on the highly processed foods.

When I was in college, I adopted a vegetarian diet for several years. However, I can tell you now that was probably the most unhealthy way for me to eat at the time. Because I was young and lacked access to the correct foods, I eliminated animals from my diet but failed to replace them with anything healthy like fruits and veggies. Instead, I opted for processed breads, nachos with cheese, chips, and candy. While vegetarian diets can be quite beneficial, you still must remember to be mindful.

## Vegan

A vegan cooking style is very similar to that of the vegetarian, though vegans will not consume any animal products whatsoever. This means no dairy, no eggs, and even no honey for some. Vegans eat a plant-based diet, meaning fruit, veggies, legumes, and grains. Anything that can be grown in the earth will be consumed by vegans.

The vegan lifestyle is one most closely associated with the principle of *ahimsa*. Many vegans take their diet choices one step further and choose not to use or wear any animal products in addition to not eating them.

## Ayurvedic

The Ayurvedic eating style is based on the ancient Indian system of medicine. In general, this way of eating involves the six tastes—which means you eat sweet, salty, sour, pungent, bitter, and astringent foods. Those who follow an Ayurvedic diet also believe in eating the colors of the rainbow.

However, the biggest guiding principle of Ayurvedic eating is based on one's unique mind-body type. There are three mind-body types in Ayurveda:

KAPHA: Typically the largest body type. Kapha types tend to be very loyal. It is recommended that they reduce oils and fats, sweets, and salt due to sluggish digestion. Instead the focus of their diet should be on spices and eating lots of veggies and high-fiber foods.

PITTA: Medium build, muscular. Pitta types tend to be focused and ambitious. They should avoid hot spices, alcohol, coffee, vinegar, and acidic foods. They should consume sweet, juicy fruits like mangoes and melons and lots of veggies with high water content—cucumbers, lettuce, and kale should be the focus of their diet.

VATA: Most slender body type. Vata types tend to be creative and enjoy change. They should avoid dry, crunchy foods; carbonated beverages; and cold, raw veggies. Warm foods—soup, cooked cereal, nuts, cooked veggies, and hot milk—should be a big part of their diet.

If after reading these you are curious to find your exact body type, there are many Ayurvedic quizzes online that can help you determine your constitution.

## Raw Food

Raw foodists believe that cooking food destroys essential enzymes. Those following the raw food diet eat uncooked, unprocessed, and mostly organic foods. This includes raw fruits, veggies, nuts, seeds, and sprouted grains.

The food can be cold or a little warm as long as it doesn't go above 118 degrees. Raw food followers will sprout seeds and beans instead of consuming them whole and uncooked. Some raw food followers will eat unpasteurized dairy, raw eggs, raw meat, and raw fish. There are four types of raw food eating:

**RAW VEGETARIANS:** Only animal products consumed are eggs and dairy.

**RAW VEGANS:** No animal products—most food is raw.

**RAW OMNIVORES:** Both plant and animal foods are mainly raw.

**RAW CARNIVORES:** Meat products are eaten only raw.

## Acid Alkaline

The principle behind the acid-alkaline way of eating is to help your body control its pH through diet. The theory is that if you're constantly putting acidic foods like red meat in your body, your system has no time to do anything else but work to remove them. In the acid alkaline diet, if you keep putting your pH at a low level, then you can cause long-lasting acidity. Those that eat the acid-alkaline way are trying to balance their pH and get it out of the acidic zone.

The general rule of thumb for the diet is 80 percent of what you eat should be alkalizing foods and 20 percent should be acidizing. Acid-alkaline followers eat mostly fruits and veggies, nuts, seeds, legumes, soybeans, and tofu. Dairy, eggs, meat, most grains, and processed foods are on the acidic side and should be avoided. Many followers of this diet also avoid alcohol and caffeine.

# Eating Habits While Practicing the Poses

So far, this chapter has discussed the benefits of nutrition in the context of yoga practice. When it comes to nutrition, you want to find the perfect system for you. Pay attention to what you eat and be aware of how you feel before, during, and after practice, then take note of what works and what doesn't. This will help you find the right way to eat for your yoga.

There are some more immediate considerations when practicing the poses. Namely, take the time to create some beneficial eating habits.

## Establishing Good Eating Habits

Here are a few common tips on what and how to eat before practicing asana:

**DON'T EAT BIG, HEAVY MEALS BEFORE PRACTICING, ESPECIALLY IF TWISTING.** You want to wring out the toxins, not your spaghetti.

**DON'T EAT RIGHT BEFORE YOU PRACTICE.** You want the food in your body to be properly digested.

**DON'T DRINK ALCOHOL BEFORE PRACTICING.** While it may give you confidence and make you feel uber-flexible, your balance and equilibrium will be off. Because your inhibitions are lowered, you may push yourself too far and cause injury.

If you're very hungry right before you practice, try eating a piece of fruit and a handful of nuts or a small snack that's easily digested.

## Eating Mindfully

There are several common methods that devoted yoga practitioners might use to prepare or bless their food, in order to eat in a more conscious manner. They are as follows:

TAKE A MOMENT TO RECOGNIZE THE FOOD IN FRONT OF YOU. Acknowledge the sustenance and good health the food is about to provide you.

TAKE A MOMENT TO CHECK IN WITH YOUR BODY BEFORE YOU EAT. What do you need in this moment to sustain good health? With yoga you've learned to move and breathe mindfully; why not eat mindfully, too?

EAT CONSCIOUSLY. Chew slowly. Try not to shovel the food into your mouth.

EAT IN A RELAXING ENVIRONMENT. Do not eat while distracted. Turn off the TV. Put away your cell phone and step away from the computer.

SERVE FOOD GRACEFULLY. The act of serving others is a good thing for your mind and your body. Connect with others as you eat your meals.

PREPARE FOOD WITH LOVE AND CARE. Think about who will be eating the food and the kind of love you want to send to them, even if it's just you—you deserve love, too.

TAKE A MOMENT TO BE GRATEFUL. This can be a prayer, grace, a blessing, or a moment of silence. Do what feels right to you.

Above all else, stay present, and healthy eating will find its way to you. Think of this as a form of meditation, which is the topic of the next chapter.

# CHAPTER SIX

# MEDITATION

Before you skim past this section because the idea of meditation sounds too far out there for you, let me tell you a little secret. If you've been practicing the poses or working on *ujjayi* breathing, you've practiced meditation.

As you might remember from the beginning of this book, yoga was broken down into eight different principles. One of these areas was meditation, or *dhyana*. This was the last limb in Patanjali's *ashtanga* before one would reach *samadhi*, or the highest state of being where the mind and body are fully merged.

Everything you've worked on up until this point has been leading you here, and now it's time to begin a meditation practice. This does not mean that you have to run off to some foreign land and commit to a vow of silence; in fact, it can be quite the opposite. You can practice meditation through walking or doing the poses. A more traditional meditation involves sitting comfortably and closing your eyes for a few minutes or an hour. Like other aspects of yoga, in meditation you are looking for what works for you.

# The Purpose of Meditation

Meditation is meant to calm the mind, but not in the way that you might think. Many people believe meditation is a tool to tune out, while in fact it is actually a tool to tune in. It's a way to train your mind and, by proxy, your body to tune in to its needs. It helps you find an inner peace that lets you operate in this world without all the anxieties and stresses that come from your daily life. It lets you leave behind fears, doubts, and the voices in your head that say, "You are doing this wrong. You are not enough. You can't do that. You won't do this." Meditation allows you to tune out those voices and tune in to the one true voice—your own.

Meditation also leads you to the now—that state of being where you're not worrying about the future or fretting about the past. Instead, you're able to concentrate on the moment and live without distractions. Meditation quiets the "me" center of the brain and allows you to be more present. It is simply the practice of continuously focusing all your attention on one thing in order to calm the mind and become inwardly aware.

# Benefits of Meditation

Just as yoga has a multitude of benefits, so does meditation. Numerous medical studies have been done on the effects of meditation on the brain. The findings range from augmenting the amount of gray matter to reducing anxiety to improving concentration and increasing happiness.

Meditation can be practiced in a variety of ways. You can do it for a minute a day or hours on end. As with the poses, there is no need to rush into meditation. Let your mind wander as many times as you want. As long as you keep coming back to a singular point of focus, you're meditating. Over time, the practice will get easier and you'll start to see the benefits in your daily life.

# How to Meditate

You don't need much to begin your meditation. As long as you've got a brain and can breathe, you're all set, but here are a few more factors to take into consideration as well:

PLACE: Find a spot in your home where you will not be disturbed. This can be the same spot you've been practicing the poses in or somewhere entirely different. As long as you can close your eyes and focus without interruption, any spot will work.

TIME: The body is most relaxed in the mornings and evenings. Many people will meditate during these times, because they find it easier to hold focus. However, if this does not work with your schedule, pick a time that makes sense to you and stick to it.

BODY POSITION: When meditating you want to be comfortable yet stay awake. Many people find that sitting up straight in Easy pose or sitting against a wall on a blanket or bolster works great for them. However, if you are ill or have a medical condition that does not allow this, then by all means lie down.

THOUGHTS: Your mind is going to wander, and that is normal. When this happens, just let the thoughts be. Don't put any judgment on them or try to change them. Let them pass and bring your attention back to the breath or the point of focus that is established in the meditation.

BREATH: Focusing on the breath is a great way to stay in the present. However, the breath in meditation is not meant to be forced or controlled. Notice your breath as it is and observe.

LENGTH AND FREQUENCY: It is best to meditate daily. If you can commit to 15 minutes a day, that would be ideal. Over time your practice will increase in length, but for now just make a daily commitment, even if it's for only a couple of minutes at a time. The benefits of meditation are cumulative, so whatever you can do is going to help you achieve results.

# Beginner Meditations

Many people like to start meditating by simply focusing on the breath, because it is the most available tool to everyone. Start simply with the breath right here as you're reading:

✦    Bring your awareness to the breath without trying to change it.

✦ Let your mind wander if it is inclined to do so, but
bring your focus back to the breath.

✦ Allow this process to continue over and over again:
focus on the breath; when the mind wanders, come
back to the breath.

✦ Do it all again.

Over time, and with practice, the mind stops wandering
as often. You'll tune in to your own voice and let any echoes
of doubt and despair disappear.

The meditations described next in this chapter will use
some version of this breath work. You are welcome to stop
here and continue to practice the poses and breathing.
However, if you choose to move on, you will find these five
beginner-level meditations to get you started:

1. Savasana meditation

2. Breathing meditation

3. Mantra meditation

4. Mindful Body meditation

5. Loving meditation

# Savasana Meditation

*The purpose of Savasana, or the final resting pose, is to let the body absorb all the benefits of the poses that you just completed. While in this resting state, it is an opportune time for you to begin a meditation practice. Because you've already established that you will end every one of your physical practices with Savasana, this is a great place for you to start working on your meditation practice.*

*Follow these steps to practice the Savasana meditation.*

1. Come into Savasana. Situate your body so that you are comfortable and relaxed. Use props if necessary. A pillow or bolster under your knees is great for relieving any back pain or giving your body extra support.

2. Close your eyes.

3. Take a deep breath in through your nose, fully expanding your ribs and your belly; open your mouth and exhale it all out.

4. Begin to breathe normally. Do not try to change or control your breath. Just let it be.

5. Scan your body and make sure every muscle is relaxed. Let the weight of your body sink into your mat.

6. Once your body is fully relaxed, bring your attention back to your breath. Observe the inhale and the exhale.

7. As other thoughts pop into your head or your mind wanders, bring your focus back to the breath.

8. Anytime the mind wanders, come back to the breath. Continue to do this for at least five minutes.

9. When you are finished, start to deepen your breath. Wiggle your fingers and your toes. Extend your arms overhead and point your feet, as if you are waking up for the first time that day.

10. Gently make your way up to a comfortable seated position.

# Breathing Meditation

*We've touched on the breath at the beginning of this section. The Breathing meditation tunes in further to intricacies of the breath.*

*Follow the instructions below to practice the Breathing meditation.*

1. Start in Easy pose or any other seated position that is comfortable. Use props if necessary to support your body.

2. Close your eyes and take a few moments to just be. Notice what you are experiencing in this moment—sounds from outside, aches in the body, thoughts of the past or future, your feelings. Do not try to do anything about them. Simply take note that they are there as you settle into the practice.

3. Bring your attention to your breath. Do not try to change it. Just observe. Notice each part of the breath. Pay attention to the details of the breath, how your nostrils expand as you breathe in, how your lungs and ribs move in rhythm, how the breath floats through your throat, how the air exits the body, and how it comes into the body.

4. Let the small movements that occur in your body as you breathe be your point of focus.

5. Continue to focus on the intricacies of the breath. If the mind wanders and other thoughts pop into your head, simply return to focusing on the movements of your breath. Keep repeating this as necessary.

6. As you maintain the focus on the breath, let everything else remain in the background—thoughts, emotions, bodily sensations—these things will come and go automatically. Let them be and keep the focus on the movements of the breath.

7. When you are finished, gently open your eyes.

# Mantra Meditation

A mantra *is a chant that supports meditation. Mantra meditation continues to focus on the breath, but you're going to add a mantra to help hone in on the present moment. This is a great meditation to practice when you're feeling overwhelmed with a giant to-do list.*

*Follow these steps to do Mantra meditation:*

1. Come to a comfortable seated position. Again, use whatever props are necessary to support your body and allow it to relax.

2. Close your eyes and relax your shoulders.

3. Take a deep, cleansing breath to fully fill your lungs and belly, then exhale and let it all go.

4. Let your breath come back to its normal rhythm.

5. Start to observe the breath. Take note of the intricacies of the inhale and the exhale. Continue to do this for several minutes. If the mind wanders, come back to focusing on the breath.

6. Now you're going to add a mantra to each breath. The words of this mantra will be your focus.

7. Observe the breath coming into the body as you silently say, "I."

8. Follow the breath as it exits the body, silently saying, "Am."

9. Observe the breath coming into the body as you silently say, "Here."

10. Follow the breath as it exits the body, silently saying, "Now."

11. Continue to focus on the breath and the words as you repeat the mantra: *I am here now.*

12. Anytime you notice the mind wandering, come back to the breath and whatever word you are on in the mantra.

13. Try to do this for at least five minutes.

14. When you are finished, repeat the full mantra one last time and then gently open your eyes.

# Mindful Body Meditation

*This meditation is great for tuning in to the body and its needs. This is a great complement to your physical yoga practice and helps unite the mind and the body.*

*Follow these steps to practice the Mindful Body meditation:*

1. Start in Easy pose or any other comfortable seated position.

2. Close your eyes and relax your shoulders.

3. Start to bring your attention to the breath. Become aware of all the intricacies of the inhale and the exhale.

4. Whenever the mind wanders, come back to the breath. Do this for a couple of minutes.

5. Shift your awareness to your body. This will be your point of focus, so anytime your mind wanders, come back to the body.

6. Scan your body from the top and move your way down. Take time at each step to really tune in to the subtle movements and feelings in each body part.

7. Observe the scalp and the top of your head. What are you feeling? Is your hair pulling on the skin of your scalp? Is it heavy?

8. Check what's happening with your forehead? Is it scrunched in or relaxed? Is the skin around your eyes heavy?

9. What about your cheeks? Are they puffed in a smile or relaxed?

10. Your jaw? Are you clenching your teeth?

11. How about your tongue? Is it resting away from the roof of your mouth, or is it swirling all over?

12. How about your throat? Can you feel the breath moving in and out? Is your neck relaxed?

13. Check your shoulders. Are they heavy, tight, or relaxed?

14. And your chest? Is it moving with each breath? How big is the movement?

15. What about your belly? Can you hear any sounds? Notice any distress or ease?

16. And your lower back? Is it strained or content?

17. Now your hips. Are they tight and stiff? Do you feel pain? Do you feel relief?

18. What about the tops of your thighs? What sensations do you feel there?

19. The backs of your legs?

20. Your shins? The calf muscles?

21. Are your feet flexed or relaxed? Can you feel the breath there? What else do you notice?

22. What about your toes? Are they cramped or limp? ❱

*Mindful Body Meditation, continued*

**23.** The bottoms of your feet? Are they cold? Warm?

**24.** Now notice the entire body as a whole. What do you feel? What is relaxed? What is strained?

**25.** Continue for another couple of minutes, scanning up and down your body. If you want to go longer, scan the body again, part by part, but this time start from the bottoms of your feet and work your way up to your scalp.

**26.** To finish, gently wiggle your fingers and your toes, then open your eyes.

# Loving Meditation

*This is a great meditation to bring compassion and love into your life. In practicing a Loving meditation, we always start with ourselves and then send the love out to others. There are various ways to do this meditation, simply by changing the mantra.*

*To practice the Loving meditation, follow the steps below.*

1. Start in Easy pose or any other comfortable seated position. Use any props that are necessary to help you relax and sit with ease.

2. Close your eyes. Start to bring your attention to the breath. Focus on the breath to settle into your meditation.

3. Focus in on the center of your chest, your heart center. Notice any sensations you feel there. Heaviness, happiness, joy, sadness. Observe these feelings, then let them go.

4. Continue to focus on the heart center and its movements as you breathe.

5. Pick one of the mantras below or make one up for yourself. Continue to breathe into the heart center.

+ *May I be kind and loving.*
+ *May I be happy.*
+ *May I be healthy.*
+ *May I be at peace.* ❱

*Loving Meditation, continued*

6. Inhale and silently say one of the mantras.

7. Exhale and imagine sending that mantra to yourself.

8. Continue to repeat this mantra, focusing on sending love to yourself with each repetition.

9. Next, picture someone in your life to whom you want to send love. This can be someone you care for deeply, or it can be someone who challenges you. Focus in on them.

10. Begin the mantra, only this time instead of saying "I" say "you." Inhale and silently say one of the phrases below.

   ✦ *May you be kind and loving.*
   ✦ *May you be happy.*
   ✦ *May you be healthy.*
   ✦ *May you be at peace.*

11. Exhale and send the mantra out to that person.

12. Continue to repeat this mantra, focusing in on sending love and kindness to the person in your thoughts. Repeat this process with as many specific people as you want.

13. Focus on sending love to the entire planet. Inhale and silently say one of the following mantras.

✦   *May everyone be kind and loving.*

✦   *May everyone be happy.*

✦   *May everyone be healthy.*

✦   *May everyone be at peace.*

14. Exhale and send this mantra out into the world.

15. Continue to repeat this mantra, focusing in on love and kindness for all.

16. At the end, come back to yourself. Repeat the mantra once more, using "I." Then gently open your eyes and go back to your day.

—

Now that you know a lot about yoga, it's time to hone in on what you need and want from the practice. Perhaps you've been working on the poses or you've started meditating. Maybe you've only read everything and are still trying to figure out how yoga fits into your daily life. Wherever you are with this practice, that is okay. The next and last chapter is designed to help you customize your experience with yoga.

CHAPTER SEVEN

# YOGA FOR YOU

Almost every day I discover something new about yoga. One day it's the fact that I can balance in poses I never thought possible, and the next it's how I handle an argument with a friend. Yoga has been like a good parent, never giving up on me, loving me unconditionally, pushing me to be my best, and constantly there when I need it.

Like any good practice, yoga and its benefits are constantly evolving. The type of awareness that yoga encourages is what allows your experience with the practice to change over time, based on what you do and don't need. Once you make yoga a part of your life, it's there to stay. This is true if you're a newly expectant mother; suddenly overworked and stressed beyond belief; or training for a marathon. No matter what, you can find a yoga practice that works for you.

# Yoga for All

There are many yoga specialties out there. These are some of the more common ones:

- ✦ Pregnant women

- ✦ Athletes

- ✦ Stress relief

- ✦ Over 60

- ✦ Injuries

If there is something specific that you're struggling with or you want to expand your knowledge of the practice in a different way, do some research and find a yoga specialty that speaks to your life situation specifically.

## Yoga for Pregnant Women

Yoga is a great way to prepare your body for the upcoming birth of your little one. However, there are many changes occurring in your body at this time, and you will need to adapt your yoga practice in a variety of ways to accommodate the pregnancy.

If you have recently become pregnant or you become pregnant after you've been practicing yoga for a while, seek out a prenatal yoga class where the teacher is well versed in the modifications you will need to make at every step of your pregnancy.

However, if you feel the need to move before you are able to get into a prenatal class, here are a few modifications you can make on your own. Do not practice deep twists while pregnant and avoid lying on your belly once you begin to show. Also, beware that the hormone relaxin is being released into your body to soften connective tissue. This is meant to make expansion of the pelvis possible; however, the hormone affects all other tissues in your body as well and can make you hypermobile, thus making it easy to over-stretch. One of the key things to remember while pregnant is to not overdo anything and, as always, listen to your body.

## Yoga for Athletes

Yoga is a great complement to athletic activities. Whether you're a marathon runner, triathlete, golfer, skier, surfer, or anything in between, yoga can help you prepare for your sport in a variety of ways. The physical postures will provide you with balance, core strength, and flexibility, but the mental aspect of yoga helps you hone in on your goals.

If you are an avid athlete, I highly recommend spending some time searching online for a program that works for your sport. I will also say that a variety of basic "yoga for athletes" classes are popping up all over. These classes focus on stretching the most commonly tight muscles in athletes and building core strength, without all the Sanskrit and philosophy. These are great classes to seek out if you are looking to add yoga to your training program but aren't necessarily looking for the meditative aspects of the practice.

## Yoga for Stress Relief

Yoga is great at relieving stress. The simple act of moving your body can release much stress, but so does meditation. A combination of these two is great for calming the mind and letting go of all your worries.

The daily poses in chapter 2 are great ones to use individually or together to help you relieve stress. Personally, I think Legs up the Wall works the best to relieve stress; however, I suggest that you experiment with the poses and meditations in order to find the perfect combination that works for you.

If you are looking for a relaxing practice outside of your home and this book, I would also recommend checking out a Yin yoga or Restorative class. These are two types of passive classes that are great at relieving stress. Yin yoga focuses on holding stretches for long periods of time to relieve tension in the muscles and joints. Restorative focuses on many different ways to relax the body. I had a teacher once describe a Restorative class as "how many different ways can we find to lie down." A Restorative class is perfect to attend after a long and stressful week.

## Yoga for Those over 60

Yoga can be adapted to accommodate many of the changes that occur in your body as you age. These accommodations may be as simple as adding props for the poses, or they can be more involved based on the current condition of your health.

If you are over 60 and just beginning a yoga practice, I recommend you seek out classes specifically meant for beginners or look for teachers who teach a program called "Prime of Life yoga." This type of yoga is aimed at those in your age group and will help you find the perfect alignment for your body.

## *Yoga for Injuries*

If you are injured, I highly suggest that you ask your doctor about what yoga programs work for you and your specific injury. There are many types of yoga out there, and while yoga can be great for aiding the healing process, if done in the wrong manner, it could exacerbate your injury. The biggest thing to remember in yoga is that if it is causing pain, then stop doing what you are doing. Yoga is not about "no pain, no gain"; in fact, it's the opposite. You want to avoid pain to gain the benefits of the practice.

As you start to figure out what specific needs you have with your yoga practice, you'll want to keep in mind that nothing is perfect, and this is a practice. There will be a lot of trial and error before you understand what works best for you.

# Advice for Beginners

Beginning a yoga practice can be very exciting. But there are many things new students do when they rush into yoga that do not serve them in the end.

Here's some advice to help you have the best experience possible as a new yogi:

TAKE YOUR TIME. You might be in a hurry to touch your toes, so you're pushing as hard as you can to get there. Maybe you're breathing through extreme pain. Avoid overdoing it so you can protect yourself against injury. There is no need to rush in yoga. It is not a competition, and there is no end goal. Yoga is a practice, and with time you will get there.

**STRIVE FOR A PERFECT FEELING INSTEAD OF PERFECT POSES.**
Yoga is all about practice, not perfection, especially when you're a beginner. While you're learning the poses, don't worry about what you might look like in a mirror; focus on how you feel in the moment. Do you have the right combo of relaxation and strength? Are you forcing the pose? Are you concentrating on your breathing?

**REMEMBER TO BREATHE.** This is a difficult one to do, but the more you can concentrate on finding a nice, steady, even breath, the easier it will be for you to get into the poses and find that perfect feeling. Also, forgetting to breathe is a big indicator that you're pushing yourself too far. If this happens, back out of the pose enough so that you can return to your breath.

**STOP COMPARING YOURSELF TO OTHERS.** Keep your eyes on your own mat. Focus on yourself. Don't try to keep up with the person next to you or the video you found online. This is your practice, and it's not meant to look like anyone else's.

**MORE IS NOT ALWAYS BETTER.** Stick to a pace that works for you. Practice *tapas* to create positive changes in your life and *svadhyaya*, the act of self-study, to find what you need to improve. Pushing too hard is never good. Again, the idea of "no pain, no gain" does not work in yoga. Listen to your body; don't push it to a place it is not meant to go yet.

**CLEAR NEGATIVE THOUGHTS FROM YOUR HEAD.** Get rid of the voice that says, "I can't do this" or "I'll never do this" or "I'm not good at this." If you are on your mat and you've showed up to practice, then you can do this, you will do this, and you are good at this.

**EMBRACE YOUR EMOTIONS.** Welcome any feelings that come over you in practice. It is not uncommon to start crying in yoga. If this happens to you, don't try to stop it—just let the tears fall. Yoga can be a huge release, but only if you let it. If you stifle your feelings or bury your emotions, you will be missing out on some of the key benefits of the practice.

**KNOW WHAT YOU WANT FROM YOGA.** Don't let anyone else's ideas influence you. A yoga practice is a personal practice. Use the idea of *svadhyaya* to find what works for you and then stick to it.

**ASK FOR HELP WHEN YOU NEED IT.** If you begin to take public classes, stay after class and ask the teacher to help you with anything you find confusing. If you're at home, get online and look for videos or seek out teachers who can answer your questions.

**TAKE YOUR TIME IN SAVASANA.** This is your final resting pose, and it's meant to be a rest to help your body absorb all the wonderful benefits of the practice. If you rush it, you miss out on so much. This goes for practicing in your own home and also in public classes. Never come out of the final resting pose and pack up your stuff before the teacher has gotten you out of Savasana. This not only short-changes you but also disturbs the students around you.

Overall, do not fret if you make a mistake. You're human, and it will happen. Simply remember to practice *ahimsa* and don't beat yourself up about it. Enjoy the ongoing process of learning.

# Looking for a Class

Even though you're probably full of information on yoga, meditation, the poses, the practice, and philosophy, you still might find yourself wanting more. In this case, consider branching out. Seeking out a yoga teacher or a class locally should be an exciting step in your practice. It will help you deepen your understanding of yoga and further your knowledge of the poses.

Public classes can be amazing, especially when you find the right one. However, they can be intimidating, especially for newer students. That's why I want to give you some helpful tips on what to do the first time you go to a public class.

## What to Bring

Bring your mat and possibly a towel and water bottle. If you do not have a mat, most studios will have one you can either rent or borrow. The studio will provide any props you might need, so don't worry about bringing blocks, a strap, or anything else.

## What to Wear

Wear appropriate yoga clothes. This should be something you feel comfortable moving in but does not slip off your body or become see-through when bending over. You want to feel good in whatever you're wearing, but it should not take you hours to find the perfect outfit. The clothes you wear should support the practice you're doing, not distract from it.

## What to Expect

It is best to show up to a new studio 10 to 15 minutes before your class. That way you can sign any release forms that are required and the receptionist or teacher can show you around the studio. Remove your shoes before entering any yoga room. Some studios require you to remove your shoes at the front door, and some have you leave your shoes just outside the yoga room. Look around to see what others are doing or ask if you're not sure of the studio's policy.

## What to Do

Once in the studio, relax and don't worry about the others around you. Everyone was a beginner once, so any nervousness you might feel is normal and no one is judging you.

Set up your mat in a place that you feel comfortable. I would suggest the center of the room in the middle row, that way you can see the teacher easily, but also the students in front of and behind you. This will help you learn visually.

Next, sit quietly on your mat and wait for class to start. You can sit in Easy pose or lie on your back, whatever feels most comfortable. This is not the time to show off the fact that you can touch your toes or balance in Tree pose. You may see other students doing what looks like a warm-up but almost all teachers are frustrated by this activity. Teachers have a class plan mapped out before they come into the room. If someone's stretching out a part of their body that needs to be strong and tight for the teacher's plan, that student is counteracting what the teacher has planned for the class. If a warm-up is necessary, your teacher will provide it within the context of the class; you do not need to do anything extra.

## What to Say

If you have any injuries that the teacher should know about, introduce yourself to him at the beginning of class and tell him your concerns or restrictions. You can also tell the teacher you're new as well. This will help you get a better class experience. Also, if you have any questions that arise throughout practice, feel free to talk to the teacher after class as well. It is best to stay quiet during the class.

# Finding the Right Class and Teacher

Once you feel confident going into a public class, you'll need to find a teacher and a class style that works for you. You might have to visit several classes and try out a variety of teachers before you make a decision. Don't be afraid to experiment. Most studios offer some sort of introductory offer for first-time clients. Take advantage of these offers to try out a variety of opportunities in your area. Once you find a teacher or class that resonates with you, make a commitment to go there regularly, whether it's once a week or several times weekly.

## Classes

The yoga classes in public studios vary; read the descriptions carefully or call ahead and ask the people at the front desk for their help in choosing which classes to attend. Tell them how long you've been practicing and what you expect to get out of the class. Do you need something more meditative and less focused on moving, or are you looking to challenge yourself physically? Ask as many questions as you can think of. Studios love new students, and they want you to be happy, so don't be afraid to seek information. Talk to the teachers as well.

## Teachers and Learning Styles

Teachers are meant to be your guide, and you want to choose one who makes you feel good about showing up on your mat every time. Find an instructor who teaches in a manner that you understand.

Also think about how you learn best and match your style to a teacher's method of instruction. Which of the following types of learner best applies to you?

VISUAL LEARNER: Are you a visual learner? Do you need to see someone demonstrate everything in order to grasp the concept? Look for a teacher who demonstrates often or situate yourself in the middle row in class so that you can watch those in front of you and behind you for visual cues as to what to do with your body.

AUDITORY LEARNER: Do you learn best by listening? Seek out a teacher who excels at giving verbal instructions. You want someone who doesn't just name the pose and expect you to get into it, but will describe each part of the alignment of the pose. Also look for someone who gives the subtle instructions of the breath and guides you to relax and find strength.

KINESTHETIC LEARNER: Do you learn by doing or having someone help you? Look for a teacher who is apt to give hands-on adjustments to her students. Adjustments help guide a student into the pose in the correct manner.

Of course most people don't always learn in one manner only. So if you can find a teacher that does all three of these things well, you'll be very fortunate. But above all else, find someone who makes you excited to practice yoga, no matter what her teaching style is.

## Yoga Retreats and Festivals

One of the fun things about yoga these days is that many studios and individual teachers conduct retreats all over the world. These are vacations that focus on yoga, though many add other activities, such as surfing or snowboarding. Once you start practicing in a studio, your fellow yogis become like small families. Eventually, they might turn into great travel buddies.

Many retreats exist, and finding the one that sounds the most exciting to you is just a matter of research and asking around. Perhaps your teacher is planning a retreat or some of your friends have found one online. You can also seek out one of the more renowned instructors, find them on a retreat, and meet new people while exploring the world. Or you can go to yoga festivals where many different instructors are teaching.

A yoga festival is great, because they're usually in a fun city and attract a wide variety of teachers from all over. Many of them even have music components to them as well, offering concerts and dance parties. Some of the bigger yoga festivals are Wanderlust Festival, Bhakti Fest, Hanuman Festival, and the International Yoga Festival in India, but there are many more out there if you look online.

If you're not interested in traveling to find new ways to practice yoga, stay alert to yoga events going on in your own community. With the interest in yoga growing exponentially every year, there's bound to be an event in your hometown, and if there's not, what's to stop you from planning one of your own?

The possibilities for yoga are endless; it's up to you to bring them into your life.

# Namaste

I hope by now you've found some aspect of yoga that works for you. Perhaps you have a pretty solid and steady home-yoga practice going, or maybe you've found a local teacher who you adore. Whatever you've discovered, I commend you for your success. It takes a lot to commit to yoga, but the rewards are well worth the effort.

Being a beginner can be hard at times, but it's a wonderful one-time experience. It is a place of openness and curiosity, where you're allowed to try new things, fail, fall, and laugh about it. It's like being a carefree kid again. Enjoy this moment and all the good things that come with it, and remember yoga is practice, not perfection, so have fun.

Know that the divine light in me salutes the divine light in you. *Namaste.*

*Appendix*

# YOGA POSE LIBRARY

Here is an alphabetical listing of the poses in this book for your convenience.

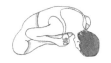

**BOUND ANGLE POSE**
*Baddha Konasana (page 46)*

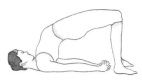

**BRIDGE**
*Setu Bandha Sarvangasana (page 120)*

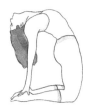

**CAMEL**
*Ustrasana (page 118)*

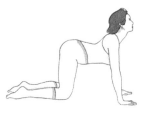

**CAT/COW**
*Viralasana (page 48)*

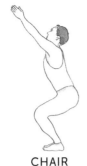

**CHAIR**

*Utkatasana (page 88)*

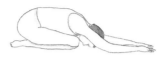

**CHILD'S POSE**

*Balasana (page 54)*

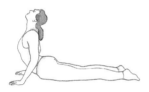

**COBRA**

*Bhujangasana (page 82)*

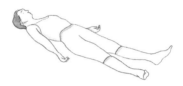

**CORPSE POSE**

*Savasana (pages 64, 136)*

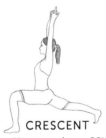

**CRESCENT**

*Alanasana (page 92)*

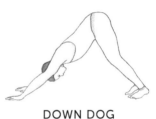

**DOWN DOG**

*Adho Mukha Svanasana (page 68)*

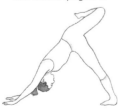

**DOWN DOG SPLIT**

*Eka Pada Adho Mukha Svanasana
(page 90)*

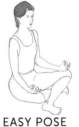

**EASY POSE**

*Sukhasana (page 42)*

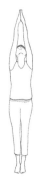

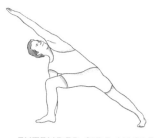

**EXTENDED MOUNTAIN POSE**
*Urdvha Hastasana (page 72)*

**EXTENDED SIDE ANGLE**
*Parsvakonasana (page 102)*

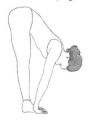

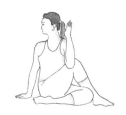

**HALF FORWARD FOLD**
*Ardha Uttanasana (page 76)*

**HALF LORD OF THE FISHES**
*Ardha Matsyendrasana (page 128)*

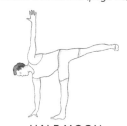

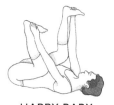

**HALF MOON**
*Ardha Chandrasana (page 106)*

**HAPPY BABY**
*Ananda Balasana (page 122)*

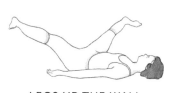

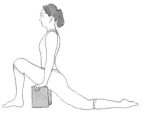

**LEGS UP THE WALL**
*Viparita Karani (page 56)*

**LOW LUNGE**
*Anjaneyasana (page 50)*

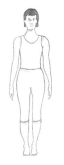

**MOUNTAIN POSE**
*Tadasana (page 70)*

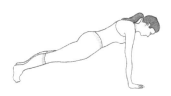

**PLANK**
*Kumbhakasana (page 78)*

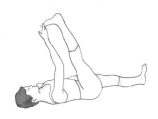

**RECLINED PIGEON**
*Supta Kapotasana (page 132)*

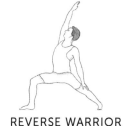

**RECLINED TWISTS**
*Jathara Parivartanasana (page 66)*

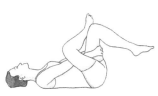

**RECLINING
HAND-TO-TOE POSE**
*Supta Padangusthasana (page 134)*

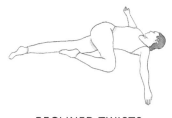

**REVERSE WARRIOR**
*Viparita Virabhadrasana (page 100)*

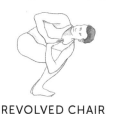

**REVOLVED CHAIR**
*Parivrtta Utkatasana (page 108)*

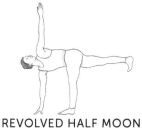

**REVOLVED HALF MOON**
*Parivrtta Ardha Chandrasana (page 112)*

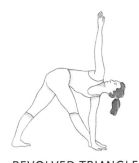

**REVOLVED TRIANGLE**
*Parivrtta Trikonasana (page 110)*

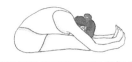

**SEATED FORWARD FOLD**
*Paschimottanasana (page 126)*

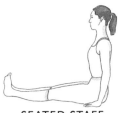

**SEATED STAFF**
*Dandasana (page 124)*

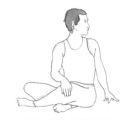

**SEATED TWISTS**
*Parivrtta Sukhasana (page 44)*

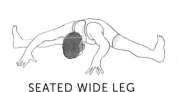

**SEATED WIDE LEG
FORWARD FOLD**
*Upavista Konasana (page 130)*

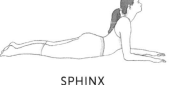

**SPHINX**
*Bhujangasana II (page 52)*

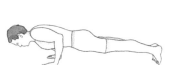

**STAFF POSE**
*Chaturanga, Four-Limbed Staff pose
(page 80)*

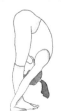

**STANDING FORWARD FOLD**
*Uttanasana (page 74)*

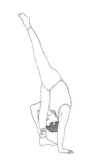

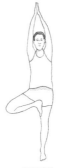

## STANDING SPLITS

*Urdhva Prasarita Eka Padasana (page 96)*

## TREE

*Vrksasana (page 116)*

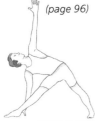

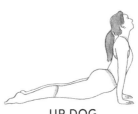

## TRIANGLE

*Trikonasana (page 104)*

## UP DOG

*Urdhva Mukha Svanasana (page 84)*

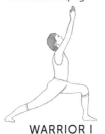

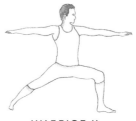

## WARRIOR I

*Virabhadrasana I (page 86)*

## WARRIOR II

*Virabhadrasana II (page 98)*

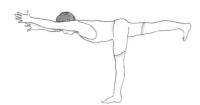

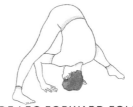

## WARRIOR III

*Virabhadrasana III (page 94)*

## WIDE LEG FORWARD FOLD

*Prasarita Padottanasana (page 114)*

# GLOSSARY

*AHIMSA*: The act or practice of doing no harm.

*APARIGRAHA*: The act or practice of nongreed.

*ASANA*: The act or practice of the physical poses or postures of yoga.

*ASHTANGA*: The eight-limbed path to yoga as described in Patanjali's *Yoga Sutras*. Also describes a specific type of yoga.

*ASTEYA*: The act or practice of not stealing.

*BRAHMACHARYA*: The act or practice of abstinence or the refrain from using excess energy.

CHAKRA: Points of spiritual energy and power in the human body.

CORE: Generally refers to muscles in the abdomen and lower back.

*DHARANA*: The act or practice of concentration.

*DHYANA*: The act or practice of meditation.

ENDORPHIN: A hormone that produces well-being.

HORMONE: A signaling molecule in the body that regulates physiology and behavior.

*ISVARA PRANIDHANA*: A devotion to god or the recognition that we're all in this together.

MANTRA: A chant that supports meditation.

**MYSORE**: A city in the south of India. It is also a particular style of teaching Ashtanga Yoga. The Mysore style allows students to practice the Ashtanga sequence at their own pace. The instructor will then work individually with each student in the room giving the students verbal instructions and hands-on adjustments.

*NAMASTE*: A traditional greeting. Translates to "the divine light in me salutes the divine light in you."

*NIYAMAS*: Describes methods of discipline.

*PRANAYAMA*: The act or practice of breathing.

*PRATYAHARA*: The act or practice of withdrawing from the senses.

*SAMADHI*: The highest state of yoga according to Patanjali. The act or practice of meditative absorption or liberation.

*SANTOSHA*: The act or practice of contentment.

*SATYA*: The act or practice of truthfulness.

*SAUCHA*: The act or practice of cleanliness.

*STHIRA*: Strength. Strong and steady.

*SUKHAM*: Relaxation. Comfortable and at ease.

*SVADHYAYA*: The act or practice of self-study.

*TAPAS*: The act or practice of working through things to create change.

*UJJAYI*: A yogic way of breathing. In *ujjayi* you breathe in a slow and controlled manner through your nose.

**VINYASA**: The act of linking the breath to movement. Also describes a set of poses that are used to move from a standing pose back to Down Dog.

*YAMAS*: Describes ways to control ourselves.

# RESOURCES

## Books

**THE YOGA BIBLE**
Christina Brown

**THE HEART OF YOGA**
T. K. V. Desikachar

**LIGHT ON LIFE**
BKS Iyengar

**LIGHT ON YOGA**
BKS Iyengar

**YOGA: THE PATH TO
HOLISTIC HEALTH**
BKS Iyengar

**YOGA SUTRAS**
Patanjali

**AUTOBIOGRAPHY OF A YOGI**
Paramahansa Yogananda

**BHAGAVAD GITA**
(various translations)

## Web Sites

**CHOPRA CENTER**
www.chopra.com

***ELEPHANT JOURNAL***
www.elephantjournal.com

**MIND BODY GREEN**
www.mindbodygreen.com

**PRIME OF LIFE YOGA**
www.samata.com

**SELF-REALIZATION FELLOWSHIP**
www.yogananda-srf.org

**YOGA DORK**
www.yogadork.com

**YOGA GLO**
www.yogaglo.com

***YOGA JOURNAL***
www.yogajournal.com

**YOGIS ANONYMOUS**
www.yogisanonymous.com

# INDEX

CPSIA information can be obtained
at www.ICGtesting.com
Printed in the USA
BVHW020342160219
540450BV00004B/9/P

9 781623 156466